AF708752

PHYSICIAN-GENERALS
IN
THE CIVIL WAR

PHYSICIAN-GENERALS IN THE CIVIL WAR

A Study in Nineteenth Mid-Century American Medicine

By

PAUL E. STEINER, Ph.D., M.D.
Professor of Pathology
School of Medicine, University of Pennsylvania
Philadelphia, Pennsylvania

CHARLES C THOMAS • PUBLISHER
Springfield • Illinois • U. S. A.

Published and Distributed Throughout the World by

CHARLES C THOMAS • PUBLISHER

BANNERSTONE HOUSE

301-327 East Lawrence Avenue, Springfield, Illinois, U.S.A.

NATCHEZ PLANTATION HOUSE

735 North Atlantic Boulevard, Fort Lauderdale, Florida, U.S.A.

This book is protected by copyright. No part of it may be reproduced in any manner without written permission from the publisher.

© *1966, by* CHARLES C THOMAS • PUBLISHER

Library of Congress Catalog Card Number: 66-12451

With THOMAS BOOKS careful attention is given to all details of manufacturing and design. It is the Publisher's desire to present books that are satisfactory as to their physical qualities and artistic possibilities and appropriate for their particular use. THOMAS BOOKS will be true to those laws of quality that assure a good name and good will.

Printed in the United States of America

H-13

PREFACE

THIS VOLUME PRESENTS a study of thirty-three physicians who became general officers in the combat services rather than in the medical department in the American Civil War. An attempt has been made to determine the significance of this phenomenon, which has not been repeated in our subsequent wars. None of these doctors became outstanding military leaders, but some were competent and moderately prominent. Nevertheless, some of them have not previously had a biography. To interpret this phenomenon as accurately and objectively as possible, the technic of using matching controls (three groups) has been used. Inasmuch as seventy-one of the total of one hundred and thirty-two officers here studied in detail was a physician, a remarkably clear picture of American medicine and medical education in the middle of the nineteenth century emerges as does the part played by physicians in the Civil War. The first six chapters are predominantly objective, the last three subjective.

In judging the quality of medicine at the time of the Civil War and the competence of these physicians, two distinct points should be considered: (a) what was the state of knowledge and the best practice at that time, and (b) to what extent was the best medicine practiced. Many medical things from that period seem primitive today, but it would be unfair to regard them as scandalous if they were in line with the foremost knowledge of that time. Unfortunately, the medical care was not always as good as it should have been, and the maximal potential satisfaction did not always accure to the military surgeon. This study presents several aspects of this situation.

ACKNOWLEDGMENTS

MANY PEOPLE HAVE GIVEN encouragement during this study and a few have been especially helpful. For the use of the records and collections in the Library of the Military Order of the Loyal Legion of the United States and for many courtesies I am grateful to Mr. J. Truman Swing and Mr. H. Durston Saylor II, Recorders-in-Chief and to Miss Stephanie Benko. Members of the military historical section at the National Archives have also given cheerfully their valuable assistance. I am deeply grateful to the following persons for biographical information: Doctor Joseph I. Waring on Doctor A. F. Anderson; Doctor James A. Waggener on Doctor Joseph G. McPheeters; Miss Pauline Duffield on General Richard Gano; Mrs. Thomas Myers Palmer and Mr. W. Harold Parham on Doctor Thomas M. Palmer; and Miss Charlotte Capers for help on Doctor Joseph R. Hill. Mr. W. Fore contributed photographic skill, and the Eleutherian Mills Historical Library helped in obtaining photographs. Mr. H. D. Milhollen of the Library of Congress gave skillful help and extraordinary interest in locating rare photographs. I am grateful to the Louisiana State University Press for permission to reproduce the photograph of General Northrop from Ezra J. Warner's *Generals in Gray*. The friends who have reviewed various chapters and criticised the ideas have my special thanks.

PAUL E. STEINER

CONTENTS

Page

Preface v

Acknowledgments vii

Illustrations xiii

Tables xv

Chapter

I. PHYSICIANS IN THE COMBAT SERVICES: STATEMENT OF THE PROBLEM 3

II. PLAN OF THE INVESTIGATION 8

III. BIOGRAPHICAL SKETCHES OF THE PHYSICIAN-GENERALS—CASE STUDIES 15

1. Major General James Patton Anderson, C.S.A. 15
2. Major General James Gillpatrick Blunt, U.S.V. 17
3. Brigadier General William Lindsay Brandon, C.S.A. . . . 15
4. Brigadier General John Bratton, C.S.A. 22
5. Brevet Brigadier General Orlando Brown, U.S.V. 24
6. Brevet Major General Cyrus Bussey, U.S.V. 26
7. Brevet Major General Robert Alexander Cameron, U.S.V. 28
8. Brevet Major General Henry Capehart, U.S.V. 32
9. Brigadier General Robert Francis Catterson, U.S.V. . . . 35
10. Brevet Brigadier General Thomas E. Champion, U.S.V. 37
11. Brevet Major General Samuel Wylie Crawford, U.S.A. 41
12. Brevet Brigadier General Daniel Dustin, U.S.V. 44
13. Brevet Brigadier General Samuel McKenzie Elliott, U.S.V. 46
14. Brevet Brigadier General John Johnson Elwell, U.S.V. . 48
15. Brigadier General Richard Montgomery Gano, C.S.A. . 50
16. Brevet Major General Thomas Maley Harris, U.S.V. . . 52

Chapter Page
17. Brevet Brigadier General David Burke Hillis, U.S.V.... 56
18. Brigadier General James Lawlor Kiernan, U.S.V...... 58
19. Brevet Major General Nathan Kimball, U.S.V........ 61
20. Brevet Brigadier General Daniel Leasure, U.S.V...... 65
21. Major General Mortimer D. Leggett, U.S.V......... 68
22. Brevet Brigadier General Charles E. Lippincott, U.S.V. 73
23. Brevet Brigadier General Benjamin Chambers Ludlow, U.S.V. 76
24. Brevet Major General William Linn McMillen, U.S.V. 78
25. Brevet Brigadier General Abram O. Miller, U.S.V..... 81
26. Brevet Brigadier General Albert James Myer, U.S.A... 85
27. Brigadier General Lucius Bellinger Northrop, C.S.A... 87
28. Brigadier General Jerome Bonaparte Robertson, C.S.A. 89
29. Brevet Major General Robert Kingston Scott, U.S.V.. 91
30. Brevet Brigadier General William P. Wainwright, U.S.V. 94
31. Brevet Brigadier General Mark Fernald Wentworth, U.S.V. 96
32. Brigadier General Edward A. Wild, U.S.V........... 99
33. Brevet Brigadier General Samuel Morton Zulich, U.S.V. 101
IV. Pre-War Life 105
Date and Place of Birth 105
Rural *versus* Urban Boyhood 105
Father's Occupation 106
Premedical Education 106
Medical and Postdoctoral Education 107
Prewar Medical Practice 108
Additional Professions or Occupations 108
Prewar Political Interest and Activity 110
Migration and Travel 111

Chapter		*Page*
	Prewar Military Education and Training	112
	Summary	114
V.	Wartime Careers	116
	Ranks and Grades Attained	116
	Length of Military Service	118
	Type of Military Service	120
	Original Rank	121
	Age at Enlistment	122
	Date of the Generalcy	123
	Duty as General Officers Prior to the Appointment	124
	Service with Negro Troops or in the Freedman's Bureau	125
	Role of Wounds and Disease	126
	Promotion Despite Disability	129
	Evidence of a Prior Medical Education	131
	Reason for Choosing the Fighting Services	132
	Military Efficiency and Distinction	132
	Crossing of Paths During the War	134
	Original Medical and Military Contributions	135
VI.	Postwar Life	137
	Date of Discharge	137
	Residual Disease and Disability	137
	Medical Training from the War Experience	139
	Return to Practice of Medicine and Teaching	140
	Medical and Other Writing	142
	Other Occupations	144
	Longevity and Death	145
VII.	Significance of Physicians in Combat Positions	147
	Weak Commitment to Medicine	147
	Poor Medical Education	148
	Undeveloped and Unattractive State of Medicine	149
	Unattractive State of Military Medicine	151
	Patriotism and Belief in the Cause	157
	Leadership in Community Affairs	159
	Personal Ambition for Military Distinction	160

Chapter *Page*

Spirit of Adventure 161

Miscellaneous Factors 164

Additional Physicians as Officers of Field Grade 164

VIII. GENERALS FROM THE OTHER PROFESSIONS 165

IX. MULTIPLE PROFESSIONS 168

Origins of the Illustrations 171

Bibliography 173

Index 191

ILLUSTRATIONS

	Page
Major General James Patton Anderson, C.S.A.	16
Major General James Gillpatrick Blunt, U.S.V.	18
Brigadier General William Lindsay Brandon, C.S.A.	21
Brigadier General John Bratton, C.S.A.	23
Brevet Brigadier General Orlando Brown, U.S.V.	24
Brevet Major General Cyrus Bussey, U.S.V.	26
Brevet Major General Robert Alexander Cameron, U.S.V.	29
Brevet Major General Henry Capehart, U.S.V.	32
Brigadier General Robert Francis Catterson, U.S.V.	36
Brevet Brigadier General Thomas E. Champion, U.S.V.	38
Brevet Major General Samuel Wylie Crawford, U.S.A.	41
Brevet Brigadier General Daniel Dustin, U.S.V.	45
Brevet Brigadier General Samuel McKenzie Elliott, U.S.V.	47
Brevet Brigadier General John Johnson Elwell, U.S.V.	49
Brigadier General Richard Montgomery Gano, C.S.A.	51
Brevet Major General Thomas Maley Harris, U.S.V.	53
Brevet Brigadier General David Burke Hillis, U.S.V.	57
Brigadier General James Lawlor Kiernan, U.S.V.	59
Brevet Major General Nathan Kimball, U.S.V.	61
Brevet Brigadier General Daniel Leasure, U.S.V.	65
Major General Mortimer D. Leggett, U.S.V.	69
Brevet Brigadier General Charles E. Lippincott, U.S.V.	73
Brevet Brigadier General Benjamin Chambers Ludlow, U.S.V.	76
Brevet Major General William Linn McMillen, U.S.V.	79
Brevet Brigadier General Abram O. Miller, U.S.V.	81
Brevet Brigadier General Albert James Myer, U.S.A.	85
Brigadier General Lucius Bellinger Northrop, C.S.A.	88
Brigadier General Jerome Bonaparte Robertson, C.S.A	90
Brevet Major General Robert Kingston Scott, U.S.V.	92
Brevet Brigadier General William P. Wainwright, U.S.V.	95

Page
Brevet Brigadier General Mark Fernald Wentworth, U.S.V. 97
Brigadier General Edward A. Wild, U.S.V. 99
Brevet Brigadier General Samuel Morton Zulich, U.S.V. 102

TABLES

Table		Page
I.	Biographical Data on the Control Generals (Group II)	9
II.	Biographical Data on the Matching Enlistees (Group III)	11
III.	Biographical Data on the Control Surgeons (Group IV)	12
IV.	Comparison of the Number of Casualties in the Four Groups	126
V.	Some Representative Physicians as Field Grade Officers—Union	162
VI.	Some Representative Physicians as Field Officers—Confederate	163

PHYSICIAN-GENERALS
IN
THE CIVIL WAR

Chapter I

PHYSICIANS IN THE COMBAT SERVICES: STATEMENT OF THE PROBLEM

In the American Civil War hundreds, if not thousands, of physicians enlisted as privates or as officers in the infantry, cavalry, artillery, and staff. Many remained in combat positions. Others transferred to the two medical departments. A third category of physicians reversed this direction, leaving the medical for a combat service. General Samuel W. Crawford is widely recognized as an example of physician become general, but he is only one among many who made the change and among thirty-three or more who reached this rank. This phenomenon reveals much about the state of medicine, military medicine, medical education, the life of physicians, and about the spirit of those turbulent times. It is the subject of this study a century after the events.

The number of physicians enrolled in combat positions is unknown. In only a few rosters in the regimental histories and the state adjutant general's reports are the men's occupation stated. The figure may approach that of the over fifteen thousand Confederate and Union military surgeons if the short term servers are included (*Brown; Memorandum*). Relative to the size of the medical and military populations, many more doctors probably had combat duty in the South than in the North. Neither the Confederacy nor the individual seceding states at first had medical organizations ready to enroll doctors proportional to the great number of volunteers. In the South, perhaps more than in the North, there was even a belief that the regimental surgeon ought to be elected, as at first were the other officers (*Wailes*). On both sides, there was early enthusiasm to enlist as it seemed the conflict would be short. Confederate Surgeon General Samuel P. Moore's problem was succinctly stated by a biographer (*Lewis*): "Many of the most capable of the younger physicians, in the ardor of the times and from various causes, sought distinction in the ranks, and as officers of commands, in the hope of more rapidly acquiring military fame." An extreme example was Captain Perrin's Company (about one hundred men) of the First South Carolina Regiment which at first contained twenty-seven physicians (*Haskell*). Even Doctor Hunter McGuire, a recent graduate, began the war as a private (*McGuire*). Some historians write of the inadequate numbers of Confederate surgeons, but many physicians were wasted as soldiers in the ranks.

Although the exact number of physician-soldiers is unknown, it was large. Many regiments had half a dozen or more (*Aten; Hart; Oates; Park; Thomas; Wailes*). Even if the average was only one per regiment, the total number would be about 2,800. From my studies, it seems probable that the figure was two to four times that value. On many occasions, it was necessary in camp or battle to detail a soldier-physician from the ranks or the line to aid or substitute for the overworked or ailing surgeons (*Barry; Crofutt* and *Morris; Delony; Hancock; Howard; Johnson; G. R. Lewis; Magee; Mulligan; Partridge; Scott; Wailes*). It seems that many regiments had one or more doctors performing non-medical duties who were available on need for such detailing. Only some of these doctors formally transferred to the medical service. Many combat physicians lost their lives, so that the figure for sick and dead doctors reported by the medical departments is below the total number. As we shall see, many of the physicians studied herein had wounds and diseases that were not reported through the correct channels for them.

In the rapid and great military expansion of 1861-1862, large numbers of officers were quickly needed. For the nearly 2,000 Federal and 800 Confederate regiments eventually organized, about 8,400 officers of field grade and 84,000 of company grade would be required for the original staffing. Eventually, about two or three times those figures would be needed as replacements. The living graduates at West Point and other military academies, and the officers trained in militia units, in the Mexican War, or in foreign armies were not nearly numerous enough to fill the need. Most of the positions were eventually filled by officers who had received their training in the war. In this scramble and competition, all men of intelligence and ability in leadership had the same chance. The physician was one of the educated members and leaders of the communities in which the troops were raised. He needed the ability to lead, brief study to learn the technical methods, and the will to forsake Medicine for Mars. Some physicians qualified and gravitated toward the top. Such doctors comprise the subject of this study.

Although a few physicians remained in the ranks, others by election or appointment became line (i.e., company grade) or field (i.e., regimental grade) officers, and some had staff positions.* Of these, a few became general officers. Among the 425 Confederate and about 1,950 Union general officers, no less than thirty-three were physicians. This figure includes six Confederate and twenty-seven Federal generals. These numbers are about proportional to the respective military populations provided those Union generals only brevetted in this rank are taken into account. There was no corresponding Confederate grade. Some of the brevet brigadier generals never actually served while they held this grade, the promotion having been made after the end of the war and pre-dated. However, nearly all of these officers had carried the responsibility of a general officer by commanding brigades while holding only a field grade commission. General officers were numerous in that war, and the story that a boy one day threw a stone at a dog on Pennsylvania avenue and hit three brigadiers might be true (*Nicolay and Hay*).

In contrast to the thirty-three physician-generals in the combat services, only two surgeons became generals in the two medical corps during the war. Assistant Surgeon William A. Hammond was commissioned the Surgeon General and a Brigadier General, U.S.A., on April 25, 1862. He was the first medical officer to reach this rank. When he was later relieved and ordered before a court-martial, he was succeeded by Joseph K. Barnes, who was awarded the same grade and rank on August 22, 1964. About ten other medical officers were brevetted brigadier generals after the war, but this list included only one volunteer (*Phisterer*). Confederate Surgeon General Samuel P. Moore carried out his duties with the relative rank of a brigadier general, but he seems not to have been formally appointed and confirmed (*Warner*).

---

*The term line officer, appropriate today, is incorrect for the Civil War period when the terminology was that here used.

Many physicians, including General Joseph Warren, chose combat duty during the Revolution (*Toner*) and in the Mexican War. However, in our wars of the twentieth century, a corresponding defection from medicine has not occurred. While a change from the medical corps to a combat service by transfer or by resignation and reenlistment would today be difficult if not impossible, a direct commissioning in the line would be possible. A study of this common phenomenon in the Civil War seemed indicated. Such an investigation, with emphasis on the etiological factors, would require biographical information on the pre- and post-war lives of the subjects as well as on their war experiences.

A study did not seem possible on the entire group of physician-soldiers for want of adequate documentation on most, and a sample might not be representative. In fact, the only entire subgroup that could be analyzed in detail was the physician-generals. Accordingly, this study has been made on the thirty-three doctors who became general officers in non-medical capacities.

It is believed that in most respects these thirty-three are representative of the entire group of physicians who served in other than medical positions; they differ in their greater military interest and ability, which led to their higher promotion.

The size of the group of physician-generals was small for statistically evaluating some factors, and the need for controls became apparent. Three groups of controls, to be described, were therefore studied in parallel. Because no significant differences were noted between the Union and Confederate groups, they were combined in the analyses. The problem was the same on both sides.

Included in the group of thirty-three physician-generals are some who had graduated from a recognized medical school and others who had practiced medicine after studying only with a physician preceptor. In 1861, there were about fifty-one recognized medical schools (*Billings*). Excluded from the group are certain generals who had studied medicine but had neither graduated nor practiced. Major General David S. Stanley, Brevet Major Generals Washington L. Elliott, James Gwyn and Marsena R. Patrick, Brigadier Generals Louis Blenker and Mahlon D. Manson, and Brevet Brigadier General George B. Dandy are among those who are excluded because, although they had some medical education, they had not graduated or practiced. Generals commissioned only in the service of a state have also been excluded. On this basis, Doctor and Major General Reuben Davis of Mississippi State Troops was eliminated. However, the problem of where to draw the line is difficult. For example, Colonel James M. Brown was killed in battle at Fair Oaks (*Stowits*). He had studied medicine in Scotland and in New Orleans and had served as an assistant surgeon in the Mexican War. Thereafter, he studied and practiced law until the Civil War. He was excluded on the basis that his commissioning as a brevet brigadier is in question.

A look at these physician-generals reveals various motives, experiences, aptitudes, backgrounds, and interests. However, certain patterns and facts emerge from the case studies which help to explain the phenomenon. The findings show why a similar situation could not occur in our subsequent wars, apart from any military regulations.

Chapter II

PLAN OF THE INVESTIGATION

THE THIRTY-THREE PHYSICIANS who became generals will hereafter be called physician-generals and designated Group I. Their geographical, social, and economic background, general and medical education, pre- and post-war medical practice and activities, extra-medical interests, and other biographical features were investigated as possible etiological factors in this phenomenon.

Three different control groups were studied and compared with the physician-generals. Each group was a matching control on one or more of the factors under study, and none was a proper control on all factors. The first is composed of thirty-three generals who were not physicians (Table I). This group is hereafter designated Group II or the "control generals." The officers selected were those whose names are alphabetically immediately subjacent to the physician-generals in the rosters of the general officers published by Miller. Thus, for the physician-general, Major General James Patton Anderson, the control general is Major General William B. Bate. As controls for Generals Brandon, Cameron, and Zulich, the names immediately above theirs in the same rosters were used. As a control for General Leasure, whose name was omitted from Miller's list, that general alphabetically nearest Leasure was adopted.

Because of the method used in their selection, these control generals match the physician-generals in rank. The mixed forces and powers that led to promotions had produced products equal in terminal grade. Military ability and achievement was one of these factors, and sometimes a major one. In these two groups, therefore, men are compared who after nearly four years had reached similar military end-points. How did their background, education, pre-war life, and military careers differ?

As the second type of control, thirty-three soldiers who had originally enlisted in the same state, rank, and position as that of the

TABLE I
BIOGRAPHICAL DATA ON THE CONTROL GENERALS (GROUP II)

Matching Number	*Name and Final Rank*	*Original Rank and Grade*[1]	*Special References*[2]
1	Major General William B. Bate, C.S.A.	Captain, Second Tennessee	Marshall; McMurray; Pollard
2	Major General W. T. H. Brooks, U.S.V.	Captain, Third U. S. Infantry	Ellis
3	Brigadier General Lawrence O'B. Branch, C.S.A.[3]	Colonel, Thirty-third North Carolina	Clark; Evans; Hassler
4	Brigadier General T. W. Brevard, C.S.A.	Captain, Second Florida	Evans
5	Brevet Brigadier General Philip P. Brown, U.S.V.	Colonel, One Hundred and fifty-seventh N. Y.	Applegate; Phisterer (N.Y.)
6	Brevet Major General James J. Byrne, U.S.V.	First Lieut., One Hundred sixty-third N. Y.	Phisterer (N.Y.)
7	Brevet Major General John C. Caldwell, U.S.V.	Colonel, Eleventh Maine	Brady; Hill; Whitman and True
8	Brevet Major General Joseph B. Carr, U.S.V.	Colonel, Second New York	Phisterer (N.Y.)
9	Brigadier General Alexander Chambers, U.S.V.	First Lieut., Fifth U. S. Infantry	Byers; Ingersoll; Lloyd; Stuart
10	Brevet Brigadier General Thomas E. Chickering, U.S.V.	Colonel, Forty-first Massachusetts	Ewer
11	Brevet Major General George Crook, U.S.A.	First Lieut., Fourth U. S. Infantry	Bourke; Reid; Schmitt
12	Brevet Brigadier General Jacob Eugene Duryee, U.S.V.	First Lieut.,Fifth New York	Phisterer (N.Y.); E. A. Davenport
13	Brevet Brigadier General A. VanHorne Ellis, U.S.V.[3]	Captain, Seventy-first New York	Phisterer (N.Y.); Weygant
14	Brevet Brigadier General Ralph Ely, U.S.V.	Captain, Eighth Michigan	Fox; Robertson
15	Brigadier General William M. Gardner, C.S.A.	Lieut. Col., Eighth Georgia	Evans
16	Brevet Major General John F. Hartranft, U.S.V.	Colonel, Fourth Pennsylvania	Bates
17	Brevet Brigadier General William S. Hillyer, U.S.V.	Private; A. D. C. (Captain)	National Archives
18	Brigadier General Rufus King, U.S.V.	Brigadier General, U.S.V.	King
19	Brevet Major General Josiah B. Kinsman, U.S.V.	Lieut. Col., A.A.D.C.	Butler
20	Brevet Brigadier General Joseph B. Leake, U.S.V.	Captain, Twentieth Iowa	Barney; Byers
21	Major General John A. Logan, U.S.V.	Colonel, Thirty-first Illinois	Mrs. Logan; Eddy; J. G. Wilson
22	Brevet Brigadier General Francis J. Lippitt, U.S.V.	Colonel, Second California	Lippitt; Orton
23	Brevet Brigadier General Peter Lyle, U.S.V.	Colonel, Nineteenth Pennsylvania	Bates
24	Brevet Major General John McNeil, U.S.V.	Colonel, Nineteenth Missouri	Blodgett
25	Brevet Brigadier General Madison Miller, U.S.V.	Captain, First Missouri	Mo. Adj. Gen.
26	Brevet Brigadier General Nathaniel Michler, U.S.A.	First Lieut., Topographical Engineers	Cullum
27	Brigadier General Richard L. Page, C.S.A.	Brigadier General	Evans
28	Brigadier General Philip D. Roddey, C.S.A.[4]	Captain, Alabama Mounted Co.	Evans; Owens
29	Brevet Major General William J. Sewell, U.S.V.	Captain, Fifth New Jersey	Foster; Stryker; Toombs
30	Brevet Brigadier General Charles F. Walcott, U.S.V.	Captain, Twenty-first Massachusetts	Bowen; Walcott
31	Brevet Brigadier General William Welsh, U.S.V.	Private, Fourth Ohio	Kepler
32	Brigadier General David H. Williams, U.S.V.	Colonel, Eighty-second Pennsylvania	Bates
33	Brevet Brigadier General George Zinn, U.S.V.	Private, Eighty-fourth Pennsylvania	Merchant

[1]Regiments are infantry unless otherwise stated.
[2]The principal general references are named in the bibliography; these are additional.
[3]Did not survive the war.
[4]Sometimes "Roddy."

thirty-three future physician-generals but in a numerically adjoining regiment were studied. These men comprise Group III and they are designated as "control" or "matching enlistees" (see Table II). The regiments used had either the next higher or the next lower number—whichever was more easily obtainable. Thus, the physician-general, Major General James Patton Anderson, who began the war as the colonel of the First Florida Infantry Regiment, was matched by George T. Ward, the colonel of the Second Florida Infantry. The reports of the state adjutant generals, the state military histories, the regimental histories, the Army Register, and other sources were used to obtain these names. Original enlistments as private were disregarded, as these men were usually not mustered in this rank, and the first commissioned grade was used instead. Group III provided an opportunity by which to compare the pre-war life and the military careers of the physician-generals with a group starting the war from equivalent positions. Since the officers of the companies and regiments at first were usually elected by the men who already knew them, in a sense this comparison is a study of men on whom community opinion was equal in the beginning.

For the third type of control, the first surgeons of the regiments in which the future physician-generals had first enlisted were used. Their names were obtained from the rosters compiled by Strait, from regimental histories, from military service records in the National Archives, and other sources. This group of thirty-three physicians is hereafter designated Group IV or as the "control surgeons" (see Table III). The physicians of this group were representative of the fifteen thousand doctors who had enlisted and, possibly, also of the younger members of the medical profession as a whole. By comparing Groups I and IV, some idea can be gained whether the physician-generals deviated from the main pattern. The future physician-general and his matching control surgeon had sometimes lived and practiced in the same or similar communities before the war. These surgeons had no opportunity or expectation of achieving military distinction or of reaching positions of leadership like those that fell to the physician-generals. They had mainly to contend with the almost endless lines of boys with the camp diseases and the clusters of wounded in the periodic battles. In what ways the mem-

TABLE II
BIOGRAPHICAL DATA ON THE MATCHING ENLISTEES (GROUP III)

Matching Number	*Name and Final Rank*[1]	*Original Rank and Grade*[2]	*Special References*[4]
1	Colonel George T. Ward,[3] C.S.A.	Colonel, Second Florida	Evans
2	Brevet Colonel John T. Burris	Lieut. Col., Fourth Kansas	Kansas Adj. Gen.
3	Colonel William N. Brown, C.S.A.	Captain, Twentieth Mississippi	Evans
4	Colonel William W. Perryman, C.S.A.	Captain, Seventh South Carolina	Dickert
5	Surgeon Josiah N. Willard	Asst. Surg., Nineteenth Mass.	Roe and Nutt; Waitt
6	Colonel Asbury B. Porter	Major, First Iowa	Iowa Adj. Gen.; W. F. Scott; Stuart
7	Brevet Brigadier General Thomas J. Brady	Captain, Eighth Indiana	Indiana Adj. Gen.
8	Surgeon Thomas S. Neal	Surg., Second West Va. Cavalry	Lang; Sutton; W. Va. Adj. Gen.
9	First Lieutenant John Pearce	Second Lieut., Fifteenth Ind.	Indiana Adj. Gen.
10	Brigadier General Friend S. Rutherford[3]	Colonel, Ninety-seventh Illinois	Illinois Adj. Gen.
11	Brevet Major General George W. Sykes, U.S.A.	Major, Fourteenth U. S. Infantry	Cullum
12	Captain Louis F. Booth	Captain, Ninth Illinois Cavalry	A. Davenport
13	Brevet Brigadier General Theodore B. Gates	Lieut. Col., Eightieth New York	Phisterer
14	Captain Edmund D. Chapman	Asst. Quartermaster (Capt.), U.S.V.	National Archives, Pension
15	Lieutenant Colonel Harvey H. Black,[3] C.S.A.	Captain, First Texas	National Archives, Service
16	Colonel John C. Rathbone	Lieut. Col., Eleventh West Va.	Lang; W. Va. Adj. Gen.
17	Lieutenant Colonel Thomas Z. Cook	Captain, First Iowa	Iowa Adj. Gen.
18	Surgeon Harvey E. Brown, U.S.A.	Asst. Surg., Seventieth New York	H. E. Brown; Phisterer
19	Brigadier General George D. Wagner	Colonel, Fifteenth Indiana	Warner, 1964
20	Captain Alexander Gillespie	First Lieut., Thirteenth Pa.	Bates
21	Brevet Brigadier General Azariah W. Doan	First Lieut., Twelfth Ohio	National Archives, Pension
22	Surgeon Orson Q. Herrick	Captain, Thirty-fourth Illinois	Payne
23	Brevet Brigadier General Gustav Heinrichs	Major, Fifth Missouri Cavalry	Missouri Adj. Gen.
24	Brevet Lieutenant Colonel Clarke McDermont	Surgeon, Second Ohio	Atkinson
25	Captain Francis G. Scott[3]	First Lieut., Eleventh Indiana	Indiana Adj. Gen.
26	Brevet Brigadier General Robert E. Clary, U.S.A.	Major, Staff, Quartermaster, U.S.A.	Army Register, 1861
27	Brigadier General Josiah Gorgas, C.S.A.	Major, Chief of Ordnance	Gorgas; Vandiver
28	Brigadier General Hiram B. Granbury,[3] C.S.A.	Captain, Seventh Texas	Evans; Mangrum
29	Major Eli J. Hickcox	Second Lieut., Sixty-ninth Ohio	Ohio Roster
30	Colonel William Searing	Major, Thirtieth New York	Phisterer
31	Lieutenant Colonel William E. Hadlock	Lieut. Col., Twenty-eighth Maine	Maine Adj. Gen.; Whitman and True
32	Brevet Brigadier General Samuel M. Quincy	Captain, Second Massachusetts	Bowen; Headley; Mass. Adj. Gen.
33	Captain Aldus J. Neff[3]	Captain, Thirtieth Pennsylvania	Bates

[1]U.S. Volunteer service unless otherwise specified.
[2]Infantry regiments unless otherwise specified.
[3]Did not survive war.
[4]For general references see the bibliography.

TABLE III

BIOGRAPHICAL DATA ON THE CONTROL SURGEONS (GROUP IV)

Matching Number	*Name and Final Rank*[1]	*Original Rank and Grade*[2]	*Special References*
1	Surgeon Thomas M. Palmer, C.S.A.	Surgeon, Second Florida	Evans; Merritt; Palmer
2	Surgeon Albert Newman	Surgeon, Tenth Kansas	Newman; Newman
3	Assistant Surgeon Joseph R. Hill, C.S.A.	Asst. Surg., Twenty-first Miss.	Evans; J. Jones
4	Surgeon Augustus F. Anderson, C.S.A.	Surgeon, Sixth South Carolina[3]	A. F. Anderson
5	Brevet Lieutenant Colonel David P. Smith[4]	Surgeon, Eighteenth Massachusetts	Atkinson; Smith; Smith; L. Warner
6	Surgeon David L. McGugin	Surgeon, Third Iowa Cavalry	McGugin; McGugin
7	Brevet Lieutenant Colonel Daniel Meeker[4]	Surgeon, Ninth Indiana	Kemper; Meeker; Russo
8	Surgeon Perin Gardner	Asst. Surg., First W. Va. Cavalry	National Archives, Pension
9	Surgeon Anson Hurd	Asst. Surg., Twentieth Indiana	Hurd; National Archives, Pension
10	Surgeon Charles Martin	Surgeon, Ninety-sixth Illinois	Partridge
11	Surgeon John J. Milhau, U.S.A.	Assistant Surgeon, U.S.A.	Army Register, 1861, Atkinson; Milhau
12	Surgeon Abner Hard	Surgeon, Eighth Illinois Cavalry	Hard; National Archives, Pension
13	Brevet Lieutenant Colonel James Norval	Surgeon, Seventy-ninth New York	Phisterer
14	Lieutenant Colonel George H. Lyman[5]	Brigade Surgeon (Major), Vols.	Keene; Lyman; Schouler; Stedman
15	Surgeon Edwin M. Shepard, C.S.A.	Surgeon, Seventh Kentucky Cavalry	National Archives, Service
16	Surgeon George C. Gans	Asst. Surg., Tenth West Virginia	Lang; Matheny; Nat. Arch., Service
17	Surgeon Nathan Udell	Surgeon, Seventeenth Iowa	Atkinson; Iowa Adj. Gen.
18	Surgeon J. Pascal Smith	Surgeon, Seventy-ninth New York	Phisterer
19	Surgeon Joseph G. McPheeters	Surgeon, Fourteenth Indiana	Maxwell
20	Brevet Lieutenant Colonel Alexander M. Speer	Surgeon, Twelfth Pennsylvania	Sipes; Spear
21	Surgeon James S. Reeves	Surgeon, Seventy-eighth Ohio	Stevenson
22	Surgeon George P. Rex	Surgeon, Thirty-third Illinois	Atkinson; I. H. Elliott
23	Surgeon Henry W. Nichols	Surgeon, Fourth Missouri Cavalry	National Archives, Pension
24	Surgeon Albert Wilson	Asst. Surg., First Ohio	McAdams
25	Surgeon Joseph S. Allen	Surgeon, Tenth Indiana	Kemper; Shaw
26	Lieutenant Colonel Richard H. Coolidge, U.S.A.[5]	Surgeon (Major), U.S.A.	Coolidge; Kelly
27	Surgeon General Samuel P. Moore, C.S.A.	Surgeon, C.S.A.	Lewis; Moore; Wickham
28	Surgeon John C. Jones, C.S.A.	Asst. Surgeon, Fourth Texas	Jones; Jones; Jones; Stone
29	Surgeon Eugene B. Harrison	Surgeon, Sixty-eighth Ohio	Harrison; Harrison
30	Surgeon Charles Newhaus	Surgeon, Twenty-ninth New York	Newhaus; Phisterer
31	Surgeon John E. L. Kimball	Surgeon, Twenty-seventh Maine	Bassford; J. M. Stone
32	Surgeon Richard H. Salter	Surgeon, First Massachusetts	Mass. Adj. Gen.
33	Brigade Surgeon Joseph H. Duffee[6]	Surgeon, Twenty-ninth Pennsylvania	Duffee

[1]U.S. Volunteer service unless otherwise specified.
[2]Infantry regiments unless otherwise specified.
[3]Originally a private.
[4]Brigade Surgeon, U.S. Volunteers.
[5]Medical Inspector.
[6]Also used name Washington J. Duffee.

bers of Groups I and IV were different before, during, and after the war were analyzed.

The four physician-generals who originally held staff appointments (Elwell, Northrop)) or positions in the regular army (Crawford, Myer) were matched in Groups II and IV by an officer holding a position as nearly equivalent as could be found.

The four groups together contain 132 officers. Groups I and IV by definition are composed of physicians. In Group III, five of the matching enlistees also are physicians because they match five members of Group I who had begun their military careers as surgeons or assistant surgeons before transferring. Thus, of the entire number to be considered, seventy-one were physicians and sixty-one had no medical education.

An attempt was made to use a fourth control group. This consisted of physicians who did not enlist in the army. One practitioner from each community represented by a future physician-general was to be used. It was hoped to determine to what extent the physician-generals were representative also of the stay-at-home civilian medical profession. It proved impossible to compile and study a matching, unbiased sample of this type, and the idea had to be dropped.

The use of any or all of these three control groups to reveal etiological and other factors is valid only if the documentation on them in the literature and records and its use were equivalent. The documentation of the military careers and lives of the officers in Groups I and II was found to be approximately equal. By definition, they were all general officers, and, as such, their principal military achievements were published in the *Official Records,* and their lives were described elsewhere. This statement applies also to those officers in Group III, the matching enlistees, who became generals. Most of the officers who did not become generals are mentioned also in the *Official Records* and other war literature. Biographical and professional information was available on some of the physicians of all groups in the medical literature as well. The biographical documentation was found to be least thorough for those members of Group III who lost their lives or resigned during the war, at a time when they had not achieved high rank or military prominence. Except for these few officers, the available data are approximately equal in the four groups as will be shown.

A biographical sketch of each physician-general is given in Chapter III. The name and some orienting data for each control officer are given in Tables I, II, and III. The standard general sources of information for the thirty-three physician-generals and the ninety-nine members of the three control groups are given at the beginning of the bibliography. In addition, special references for each control follow his name in the three tables. The *Official Records* are indispensable for their military records, and the state adjutant general's reports give additional data. The pension and military service files in the National Archives are the best source of information on their wounds and diseases. The military histories of the states (e.g., *Bates, Phisterer, Eddy, Stuart,* etc.) were also good sources of information.

Chapter III

BIOGRAPHICAL SKETCHES OF THE PHYSICIAN-GENERALS–CASE STUDIES

1. Major General James Patton Anderson, C.S.A.

PATTON ANDERSON was born at Winchester, Tennessee on February 16, 1822 (*Anderson; D.A.B.; Warner*). He attended schools in Tennessee and Kentucky. In 1840, he graduated from Jefferson College, Canonsburg, Pennsylvania. He then studied medicine and practiced at Hernando, Mississippi, an area only recently evacuated by the Indians. Here, he also studied law in an office, and was admitted to the bar in 1843. Soon, he was a deputy sheriff and a member of a local militia regiment. In 1847, he recruited a company for service in Mexico and was later elected the lieutenant colonel of the regiment, but he had no combat experience. He spent one term in the Mississippi legislature. Because of bad health beginning in 1849, characterized by "fever and ague" engendered in the miasmatic climate, he was advised to move to a dry, cold climate. Consequently, in 1853, he went to Washington Territory by way of Nicarauga as the U. S. Marshal on appointment by Secretary Davis. Here, he also took a census and prospected for gold. Elected the territorial delegate to Congress, he traveled to Washington by way of Panama in 1855. He declined the appointment by President Buchanan in 1857 to return to Washington as governor, and assumed the management of a plantation in Florida. He was an elected delegate to the secession convention in Tallahassee in January, 1861 and to the convention of Southern states at Montgomery in February. Here, he proposed that slaves should be used as the cooks, nurses, teamsters, and pioneers of the Confederate army. The idea was adopted only in part.

Anderson recruited a company in March, 1861 and became the colonel of the First Florida Regiment even before the hostilities began. By February, 1862 he was a brigadier general and two years

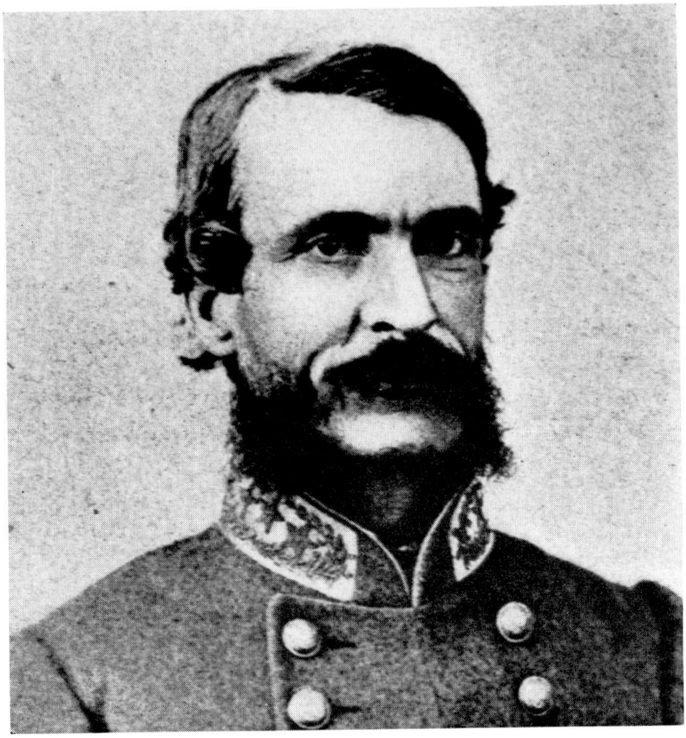

Major General J. Patton Anderson, C.S.A.

later a major general. He commanded brigades or divisions—usually as a substitute—at the great battles of Shiloh, Perryville, Stone's River, Chickamauga, and Chattanooga. After Shiloh, he was ill with "fever" for some weeks in Mississippi. In the spring of 1864, he was in charge of the district of Florida. He returned to the Army of Tennessee at Atlanta, and at the Battle of Jonesboro on August 31st he was severely wounded (*O.R. 1*). When he rejoined in March, 1865 in North Carolina, he was not yet well. Of the aggregate of 4,666 men in his division on April 17th, only 1,005 were present for duty (*O.R. 2*). He was paroled at Greensboro.

In accordance with this varied and important record, General Anderson's military correspondence is voluminous (*O.R. 3*). His reports tend to be long and detailed but unusually candid, and hence helpful to the historian. Despite his prewar political record, he seemed to keep aloof from army politics. At the restricted meeting of senior officers in January, 1864, at which General Patrick Cleburne had proposed to free the slaves willing to bear arms, he suffered painful emotions at the monstrous proposition (*O.R. 4*). After the war, he published a farm paper in Memphis and was a tax collector. He died on September 20, 1872 and was buried in Memphis.

In summary, this physician's interest in medicine was transient and superseded already before the war by law and politics. Nothing in his war record indicates he had been a physician. Something of a rolling stone, he seems not to have fully used his considerable talents.

2. Major General James Gillpatrick Blunt, U.S.V.

James G. Blunt was born in Trenton, Maine on July 21, 1826 (*Blunt; C.A.B.; D.A.B.*). From his fifteenth to his twentieth years, he was a sailor. In 1849, he graduated from the Starling Medical College at Columbus, Ohio. He practiced in New Madison, Ohio until 1856 when he moved to Greeley, Kansas with his wife and children. Here, he was drawn into the anti-slavery movement, became acquainted with John Brown, and was a delegate to the constitutional convention of 1859 at Wyandotte, while continuing general practice in a small town.

In May, 1861, Doctor Blunt enlisted as a private (*Blunt; Kansas Adj. Gen.*). Soon, he helped to recruit the Third Kansas Infantry Volunteers and was elected their lieutenant colonel, although he had no military training and was not widely known (*Castel*). His subsequent war service was limited to the then far west—to Kansas and the adjoining parts of Missouri, Arkansas, and the Indian Territory. Although he held a number of departmental, district (Department of Kansas, District of Kansas, District of the Frontier, District of the Upper Arkansas, District of South Kansas), and army (Army of the Frontier, Army of the Border) commands, his white troops—usually extended by Indians and Negroes—rarely numbered 5,000 except on one occasion when, at Prairie Grove for a few days, he led 8,000 volunteers. He was promoted to brigadier general as early as April 8, 1862 and to major general in December of that year. He was involved in many actions and engagements but in no major battle (*Blunt; O.R.Index*). His largest battle took place on December 7, 1862 when, with Brigadier General F. J. Herron, he defeated

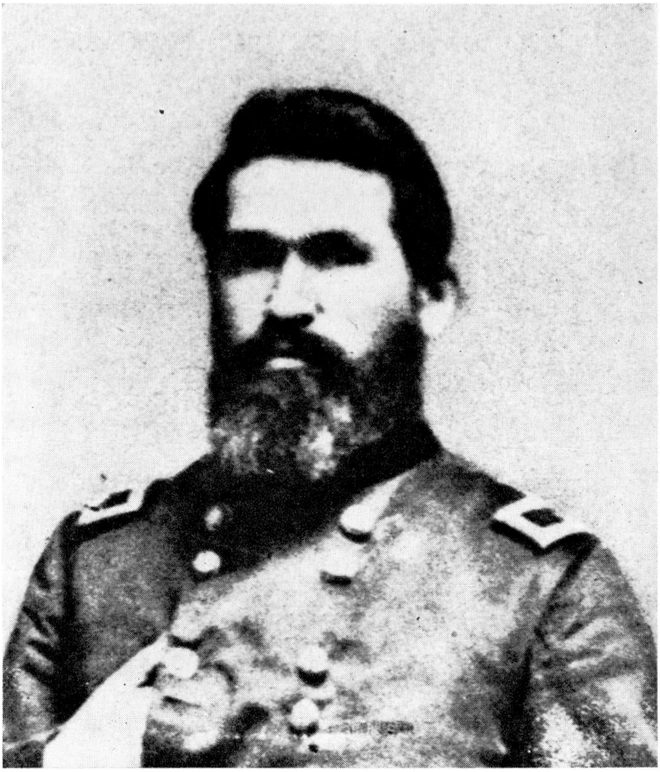

Major General James G. Blunt, U.S.V.

General T. C. Hindman at Prairie Grove, Arkansas. In this encounter, his casualties, numbering 1,251, indicate a severe action (*O.R. 5*). Most of his numerous victories, however, came in running actions against raiders, bushwackers, and guerillas such as Shelby and Quantrill in what were, essentially, police affairs. Nevertheless, he played an important part in protecting Missouri against Hindman in 1862 and Kansas against General Sterling Price in 1864 (*O.R. 6*). He penetrated beyond the Arkansas River on several occasions. His largest command, that of the Department of Kansas in 1862, included the frontier Forts Kearny, Laramie, Larned, Leavenworth, Randall, Riley, Scott, and Wise in Nebraska, Kansas, and Colorado.

The war effort in Kansas, thinly populated and a state only since

January, 1861, became deeply involved in partisan politics and a mixed fight for political influence, lucrative war contracts, and abolition. Blunt became committed to the side of General (and Senator) James K. Lane, to whose influence rather than to exceptional military achievement he owed his general's stars. General Blunt quarreled with the several governors of Kansas and with nearly all of his military superiors in the Department of the Missouri at Saint Louis, including Generals Halleck, Curtis, and Schofield. On several occasions, he carried the controversies to the War Department (*O.R. 7*) and even to the President (*O.R. 8*). At one time, Generals Blunt and Kimball quarreled over the transportation at Fort Smith; both were physicians (*O.R. 9*). But most of his caustic combativeness was directed against West Pointers. As the war went on, his influence and responsibilities gradually diminished. His successes were usually achieved by vigorous, bold, rapid and long night marches with dawn attacks, the use of deception, and a good intelligence system—all marks of native ability. However, his administration was often lax, his tactics questionable, and his talk if not actions sometimes insubordinate. Nevertheless, he was popular among certain people and he was voted a resolution of thanks by the Cherokee Nation in 1863 (*O.R. 10*).

General Blunt was described as resolute and selfconfident, but also as coarse, unscrupulous, licentious, a heavy drinker, and emotionally unstable (*Castel*). His large military correspondence in the Official Records is usually vigorous but sometimes contentious to a point that suggests paranoid trends (*Blunt; O. R. Index*). His official post-action reports are clear but they tend to magnify small events and details. His considerable ability in tactics was not matched by his strategic concepts, which were outmoded, as they were concerned mainly with taking and holding territory. The long range fate of Kansas was actually not determined there but elsewhere.

Although he carried the responsibility, there is no evidence in General Blunt's reports or correspondence that he took any unusual interest in the physical welfare of his men, that their health was better than that of other units, or that they received better medical or surgical care. He rarely mentioned his medical officers in reports. His own health was good except for a "fever" lasting for over three months (July-September) in 1863, which put him to bed for over ten days in September and kept him from the saddle even longer (*O.R. 11*).

Doctor Blunt was mustered out of the federal service in July, 1865. He practiced at Leavenworth until 1869 when, abandoning medicine for a second time, he became a solicitor of claims before various departments in Washington. Here, he came under a cloud in 1873 on a charge of conspiring to defraud the government and the Cherokee Indians, but the action was discharged in 1875. He was admitted to St. Elizabeth's hospital in February, 1879, where he died on July 25, 1881. He was buried in Arlington.

Death was attributed to "general paralysis of the insane with epileptiform convulsions" (*Nat. Arch.*). Mental disease had already been evident before Blunt moved to Washington in 1869. His judgment, insight, and memory were there impaired; he fell asleep even during conversations, made sudden irrelevant and divergent remarks, and claimed extravagant and impossible financial and medical successes. These abnormalities were recognized by Surgeon General J. K. Barnes and others, and they led to his admission to this institution, where they progressed during the years before his death. At least three physicians testified that his mental faculties became unsound in the summer of 1863 with the acute febrile illness that had interrrupted his campaign in the Indian Territory. Carried to Fort Smith in an ambulance, he was stricken both mentally and physically for weeks, with periods of delirium and unconsciousness. He was left with absent-mindedness, pain in the head, and insomnia. No diagnosis has been found for this illness.

Death at age fifty-five, after a progressive mental illness lasting at least twelve years and possibly eighteen, in the nineteenth century cannot be diagnosed today with certainty from the available information. General paresis was then a clinical rather than an etiological diagnosis, and the presence of epileptiform seizures casts doubts on its identification with the specific infection the term denotes today. Neoplasms, degenerative and vascular lesions, and chronic granulomas would all have to be considered in diagnosis.

In summary, Doctor Blunt's career illustrates the advancement of a private to general and of a physician to general. Of the three professions he practiced namely, the medical, military, and legal, medicine seems to have interested him least. All of his military career was spent in the West, mostly in the command of military districts, with mixed troops. His fatal disease might have been service-incurred.

3. Brigadier General William Lindsay Brandon, C.S.A.

William Brandon was born near Washington, Mississippi in about 1802 (*Evans; Nat. Arch.; Warner*). He was educated at Washington College and the College of New Jersey (now Princeton). He also studied medicine and was often consulted. He became a planter interested in horses and hunting, a member of the militia, and a member of the state legislature in 1826.

Brandon enlisted early in 1861 in the First Mississippi Battalion, in which he was first the major and then the lieutenant colonel. This unit went to Virginia that summer as a part of the Twenty-first Mississippi Regiment. In the battle of Malvern Hill in July, 1862, he was wounded by a grape shot and his right leg was amputated

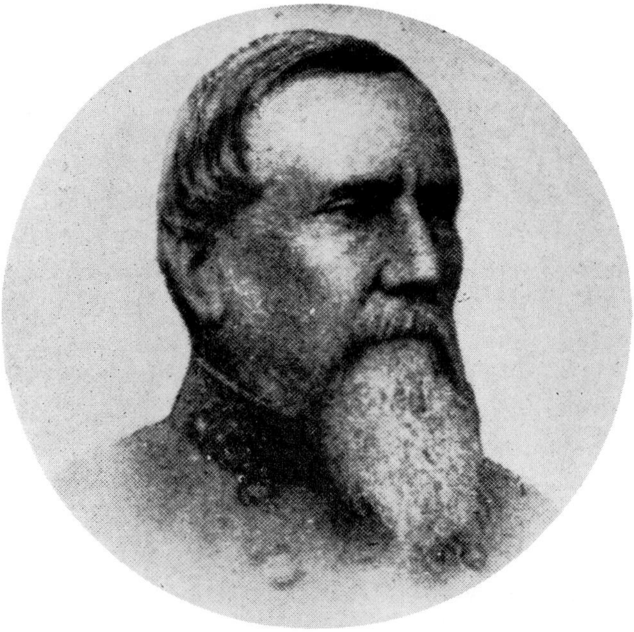

Brigadier General William L. Brandon, C.S.A.

(*Nat. Arch.; O.R. 12*) but he remained in service. After the battle of Gettysburg he was promoted to colonel. After the battle of Chickamauga he resigned, giving as reasons the poor fit of his artificial leg, his advanced age, and the recurrence of his "old disease" of 1862 from Virginia—the recurrence caused by the irritation from drinking the local lime water around Chattanooga.

However, in June, 1864, he was promoted to brigadier general and sent to Mississippi in charge of the bureau of conscription. This assignment became difficult as interest in the war waned after the state was partly cut off by Sherman. His difficulties with the governor over the jurisdiction of troops had finally to be taken to the courts (*O.R. 24, 25, 26*). After the war Brandon retired to his plantation, where he died on October 8, 1890.

In summary, this physician of uncertain medical education and part time practice served in the war as an infantry officer. He tried to resign after suffering from a camp disease and the loss of a leg in battle, but despite these handicaps and advancing age he was commissioned a brigadier general and assigned to conscription service. After the war, he lived in retirement.

4. Brigadier General John Bratton, C.S.A.

John Bratton was born at Winnsboro, South Carolina on March 7, 1831 (*Evans; Warner*). He graduated from the South Carolina Medical College in 1853 and practiced in Winnsboro. After secession, he enlisted as a private in the Sixth South Carolina Volunteers (state service), and by election was a captain at Fort Sumter. He then enlisted as a private in the Confederate service and went up through the grades to colonel by 1862. He had heavy service in Longstreet's corps of the Army of Northern Virginia and was recommended for promotion to brigadier in 1863 (*Nat. Arch.*), but this did not come until May, 1864 when he succeeded the slain General Micah Jenkins. At Appomattox, he surrendered the largest brigade (1,548 men) despite heavy losses (*O.R. 16*).

Bratton was wounded twice. As a lieutenant colonel, he was shot in the right arm, the ball entering also the body, and he was captured, both at Seven Pines (*Bratton; O.R. 17*). He later wrote of the kind care he had received from the Union surgeons and of the

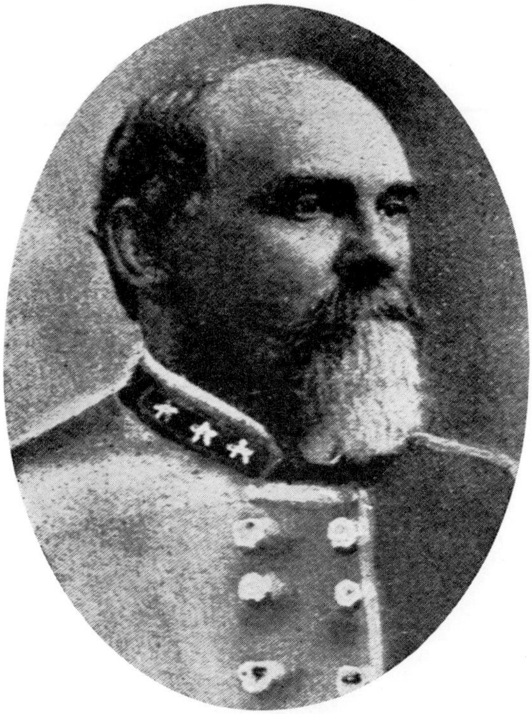

Brigadier General John Bratton, C.S.A.

special consideration shown by Generals Kearny and Birney, both strangers, neither of whom survived the war. Then, on October 7, 1864, as a brigadier Bratton was again wounded, in the engagement on the Darbytown Road, and incapacitated for six weeks (*O.R. 18*).

After the war, Bratton became a planter and politician (*D.A.B.; Warner*). He was a delegate to the state constitutional convention in 1865, a state senator in 1865-66, a United States congressman in 1884-85, a delegate to Democratic conventions in 1876 and 1880, and the state comptroller in 1881. He died at Winnsboro on January 12, 1898.

In summary, this physician entered the military service as a private before the war began, and he was a brigadier by 1864. He was wounded twice in battle and captured once. After the war, he became a planter and politician. Nothing in his war record suggests that he had a medical education.

5. Brevet Brigadier General Orlando Brown, U.S.V.

Orlando Brown was born at Groton, Connecticut on April 13, 1827 (*Brown*). He graduated from the medical department of Yale University in 1851 (*Brown, 1904*), and at Harvard in 1856 (*F. H. Brown*). He was practicing in Wrentham, Massachusetts when the war came. He was first married in 1853 and, his wife having died, again in 1855 (*Nat. Arch.*).

Doctor Brown became the assistant surgeon of the Eighteenth Regiment Massachusetts Volunteers in July, 1861 and the surgeon of the Twenty-ninth Massachusetts in December of that year on appointment by Governor Andrew (*Heitman; Mass. Adj. Gen.; Osborne; Strait*). The Eighteenth Regiment had duty in and around Washington. The Twenty-ninth helped capture Norfolk and Suffolk and then participated in McClellan's Peninsular Campaign. In July, 1862, at Harrison's Landing, Surgeon Brown became incapacitated for field service by chronic diarrhea and cystitis (*Brown, 1903*).

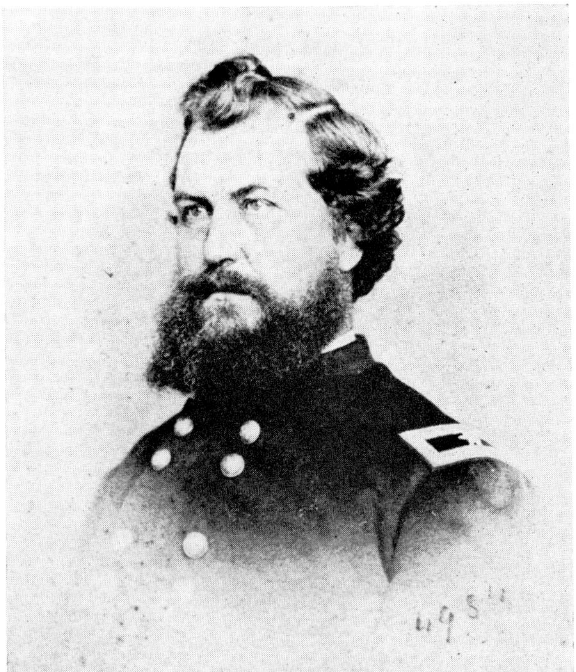

Brevet Brigadier General Orlando Brown, U.S.V.

On his application for sick leave of absence, the brigade surgeon certified that " * * this officer will die if not allowed leave of absence." But General E. V. Sumner disapproved, endorsing: "Let this officer die then and set an example of heroism to the men." Doctor Brown, consequently, resigned in July, 1862 on account of his illness. Not Surgeon Brown but General Sumner died eight months later.

On going to the rear, Brown improved enough at Fort Monroe to accept an offer as contract surgeon made by the medical director of the department. In this capacity, he helped to establish the large general hospital at Newport News and later to move it, together with a large contraband camp that had grown up nearby, to Craney Island. After fifteen months, he was commissioned an assistant quartermaster (captain) with the duty of recruiting colored troops in the State of Virginia south of the James River (*O.R. 19*). Later he became the Assistant Commissioner of the Bureau of Refugees, Freedmen, and Abandoned Lands for the area (*O.R. 20*). On June 19, 1865, he was commissioned the colonel of the Twenty-fourth Regiment U. S. Colored Infantry, organized at Camp William Penn, Pennsylvania (*Army Register*). He was brevetted a brigadier general in January, 1866 for meritorious services, and honorably mustered out in August, 1868 (*Heitman*). For some time, he was on General Schofield's staff as an acting assistant adjutant general helping to close the Freedman's Bureau.

Doctor Brown resumed practice in Washington, Connecticut. He became the president of his county medical society and of the state society in 1889. He died in August, 1904 at his home, of chronic interstitial nephritis, aged seventy-seven years (*Nat. Arch.*). He had been a genial, popular, and prominent physician at Litchfield and the adjacent area.

The reason for Doctor Brown's transfer from the medical to the quartermaster services, where he had no increase in rank, is not known. It may be related to the deal he got from General Sumner. His special duties, however, led eventually to the colonelcy of the regiment of negroes. He had had no military training or experience in action.

In summary, this case is an example of a physician who transferred from the medical department first to a staff corps and eventually to the colonelcy of a colored regiment, and it is possible that he transferred for this purpose. He did not serve as a general officer, which grade was awarded him by brevet at the end of the war, when he resumed the practice of medicine.

6. Brevet Major General Cyrus Bussey, U.S.V.

Cyrus Bussey was born at Hubbard, Ohio on October 5, 1833, the son of a Methodist clergyman (*C.A.B.; N.C.A.B.; Stuart*). The family soon moved to southern Indiana, where the boy had a meager education. From age fourteen, when he began clerking in a dry goods store, he was essentially a merchant. Before he moved to Bloomfield, Iowa, at age twenty-two as a newly-wed, he had studied medicine for two years with a brother and practiced briefly. From 1858, when he was elected to the Iowa senate, he was a

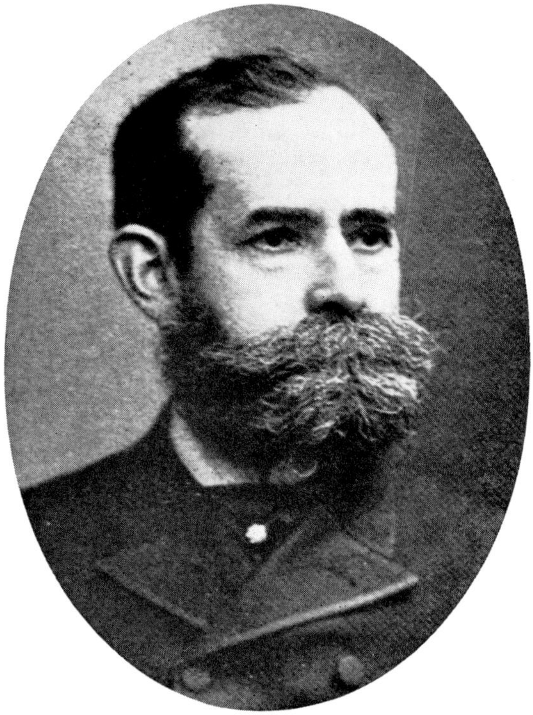

Brevet Major General Cyrus Bussey, U.S.V.

politician as well as merchant, supporting Douglas at Baltimore. With the war, he became a strong Unionist. He was described as five feet and eleven inches tall and slender; he had a fair complexion but dark hair and eyes, winning manners, ready wit, and easy conversation.

Senator Bussey was appointed an aide to Governor Kirkwood, and as a lieutenant colonel in the militia he spent the next two months guarding the southern counties against invaders. On August 10, 1861, he became the colonel of the Third Iowa Cavalry, which he had recruited. With this regiment, he came under the command of General Samuel R. Curtis in the Army of the Southwest, fighting in the Battle of Pea Ridge, Arkansas in March, 1862. Here, his regimental casualties were fifty men, eight of them scalped by Pike's Indians (*Stuart; O.R. 21*). In July, 1862, he fought under General Frederick Steele, Army of the Southwest, in the campaign in Arkansas, usually in charge of a cavalry brigade. By the spring of 1863, he reached the District of Eastern Arkansas at Helena. In Grant's campaign against Vicksburg, Bussey was briefly east of the Mississippi in the Army of the Tennessee. On January 5, 1864, he was promoted to brigadier general of volunteers. He spent the remainder of the war at Little Rock or at Fort Smith in the Department of Arkansas. The grade of brevet major general was later awarded to date from March 13, 1865.

In summary, Bussey's service was all in the cavalry or in the command of districts that were relatively quiet except for the guerilla activity. Except for a few months east of the Mississippi, all of it was in Arkansas, Missouri, or in the Indian Territory. His usual command was a brigade or a district. Although some of his service was strenuous, he was in no major battle except Pea Ridge. Militarily he appears to have been self-taught, as he was not under the direct command of a trained cavalryman for any extended period.

After the war, Bussey was in business successively at Saint Louis, New Orleans (1866-1882), and New York. He was a delegate to the Republican conventions in 1868 and 1880, and to a Methodist conference in London in 1880. In 1889, he became the Assistant Secretary of the Interior in the Harrison administration, serving until 1893 under the secretary, his former military aide. Thereafter,

Julian R Youmans M D

he practiced law in Washington, dealing with military pension claims. He died after long invalidism on March 2, 1915, and was buried in Arlington.

Although General Bussey was never wounded, he contracted several diseases and was never entirely well after leaving the army. He suffered from malaria in the swamps of Arkansas in July, 1862, at Vicksburg in 1863, and in Arkansas in August and September of 1864 (*Nat. Arch.*). He was treated for malaria many times after the war—at least as late as 1882 in New York. Following a severe exposure in February, 1862 and subsequently, he developed severe "neuralgia" and "rheumatism" of the neck and back. At one time, in 1862, he was obliged to ride along in an ambulance. In September, 1864, he had an attack of jaundice, and in March, 1865 he was quite sick with erysipelas (*O.R. 23*) . For these ailments, he had several leaves on surgeon's certificate of disability, but he remained on duty most of the time. From 1906, he was a semi-invalid with severe chest pain requiring medication. More than in the case of any other of the seventy-one physicians in this study, they suggest anginal attacks. Whatever the nature of the various illnesses, they did not greatly shorten his life as he lived into the eighty-third year.

From the nature of his service, General Bussey left a sizeable amount of military correspondence (*O. R. Index*). Nothing in these writings indicates that their author was a physician. His complaints that he found 1,000 men sick in hospitals in Helena in January, 1863, that there was room for reform, and that the public business had been extravagantly managed were not different from the observations recorded by many commanders who were not physicians (*O.R. 24*). He seems to have been naturally gifted, but, possibly, something of a rolling stone. The available evidence does not explain all of his actions. It is obvious, however, that his interest in medicine was brief and mild.

7. Brevet Major General Robert Alexander Cameron, U.S.V.

Robert Cameron was born in Brooklyn, New York, of pre-Revolutionary forebearers on February 22, 1828 (*D.A.B.; N.C.A.B.*). The family moved to Valparaiso, Indiana when he was fourteen. He at-

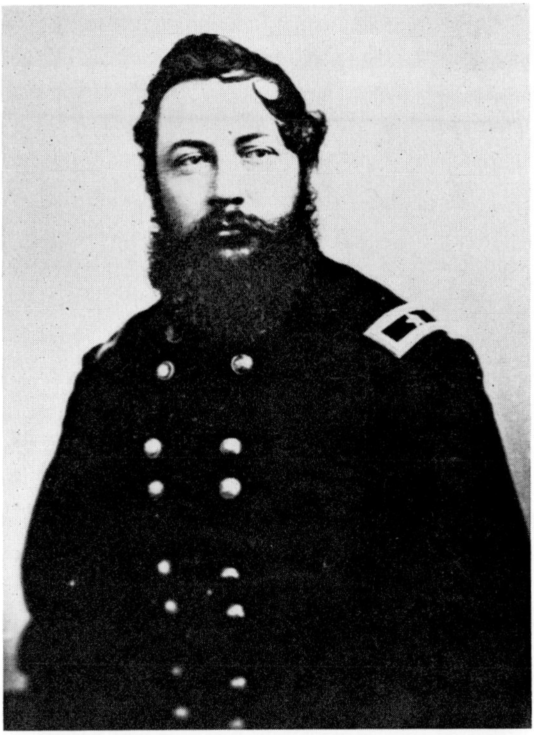

Brevet Major General Robert A. Cameron, U.S.V.

tended the public schools and graduated from the Indiana Medical College at Laporte in 1849 (or 1850), and then attended Rush Medical College in Chicago for some time. From 1851 to the war, he practiced at Valparaiso. From 1857, he also owned and published the Valparaiso *Republican*. In 1860, he was a delegate supporting Lincoln at the convention in the Wigwam, and he was serving in the lower house of the Indiana legislature.

On the first call for troops in April, 1861, Doctor Cameron raised a three-month company, which went at once to the West Virginia campaign of McClellan as a part of the Ninth Indiana Regiment with himself as captain. They were engaged at Philippi and Carrick's Ford. In the three-year service that followed, he became the lieutenant colonel of the Nineteenth Indiana Infantry in July, 1861, and the same grade in the Thirty-fourth Indiana in February, 1862;

by June of that year he was its colonel. This regiment, under General Pope, was at the fall of Island No. 10, New Madrid, and Memphis, all on the Mississippi River. In the Vicksburg campaign, they were seriously engaged only in the battle at Champion Hill. In August, Cameron was promoted to brigadier general. The basis for this advance is not clear; he had not commanded a brigade. Later in 1863, General Cameron's brigade was sent with the Thirteenth Corps to Bank's Department of the Gulf. They took part in the ill-fated Red River campaign in March-April, 1864. Here, Cameron led a small division and, after General Ransom was wounded at Sabine Cross Roads, the Thirteenth Demi-Corps (two small divisions) itself. Neither in the battle at Sabine Cross Roads nor at Pleasant Hill were Cameron's men heavily engaged, although the Corps had 1,405 casualties before he assumed its command (*O.R. 25*). In June, 1864, General Cameron was assigned to the direction of the District of La Fourche on the west bank of the Mississippi in Louisiana. The district was guarded by about twelve greatly reduced regiments, widely scattered (*O.R. 26*). The administrative load was quite large but the mission was essentially a police job. He held this position until he resigned in June, 1865. The grade of brevet major general was awarded later but ante-dated to March 13, 1865.

Doctor Cameron resumed medical practice at Valparaiso for two years, and at Phelps, New York for two more (*Nat. Arch.*). He then became a promoter of migration to the far west. As a member of a group, he helped select the sites and found the communities at Greeley, Manitou, and Colorado Springs, Colorado in 1870, and at Fort Collins in 1873. He practiced medicine at Greeley from 1870 to 1878, when he moved to Denver. Here, he was post office inspector in 1880, warden of the state penitentiary at Canon City in 1885-1887, and a commissioner of immigration for the Denver, Texas and Fort Worth Railroad after 1888. He died on a fruit farm, that he had developed at Canon City, on March 15, 1894. Three geographical features were named after him: The parish of Sabine in Louisiana changed its name to Cameron parish to compliment him; Cameron's Cone in El Paso county and Cameron's Pass in Laramie county, both in Colorado, also bear his name (*C.A.B.*).

This active life belies the state of his health. During the approach to Vicksburg in March, 1863, Colonel Cameron was invalided home under the diagnosis of "acute purulent ophthalmia" (*Nat. Arch.*). He had had to be transported in an ambulance at times. This condition led to some impairment of vision. He later claimed that the disease had been caused by material thrown into his eyes by an exploding rebel shell. Soon after returning to the field at Vicksburg, he developed a diarrhea, which followed him to the grave. He claimed that it caused piles and an umbilical hernia. From about 1892, he had severe attacks of abdominal pain in addition to the chronic diarrhea, requiring narcotics at times and causing invalidism. He was reduced to a low residue, soft diet. The physicians who attended him during the last year found at necropsy four areas of contraction and induration, each about six inches long, one in the jejunum and three in the ileum. Only fluids could pass these strictures. They were attributed to the healing of ulcers, and the cause of death was diagnosed as "chronic enteritis." Neither bacillary nor amebic dysentery ordinarily produce multiple elongated strictures in the small intestine. The description fits that of regional enteritis, first described as a separate entity in the present century. Today one wonders whether Doctor Cameron could have had this disease.

Doctor Cameron had a number of interests and medicine did not absorb his full energy. His wartime career was active but militarily not distinguished, although he ably carried out his assignments. He was engaged in only one major battle but he was near by at others. It happened that he came under the command chiefly of political generals. These included Generals Gorman, Prentiss, Hovey, McGinnis, McClernand and, later, Banks. Among his superiors, only Ransom was outstanding, but he was over Cameron for only a few weeks in 1864. For Cameron it was, then, a long hard war with much disease and little fighting. There is nothing in his voluminous military correspondence to indicate that he was a physician (*O.R. Index*). At Vicksburg his path crossed that of many others of the physician-generals mentioned in this study. At La Fourche, Doctor Lippincott, then commanding the Thirty-third Illinois, came under his immediate charge but there is no indication of mutual professional recognition. It is possible that his death resulted from the late effects of a service-incurred dysentery and that his name, like many others should be added to the mortality lists of that war. Like many other physicians, he often treated himself when ill, possible inadequately, and his service medical record is incomplete.

8. Brevet Major General Henry Capehart, U.S.V.

Henry Capehart was born in Cambria County, Pennsylvania on March 18, 1825 (*Capehart*). The details of his early life and education have not been located. When the war came, he was practicing medicine, since 1849, in Bridgeport, Ohio (*Lang*). He was described as five feet and eight inches tall, brown haired, grey eyed, and of a fair complexion (*Nat. Arch.*). His first wife died in 1854

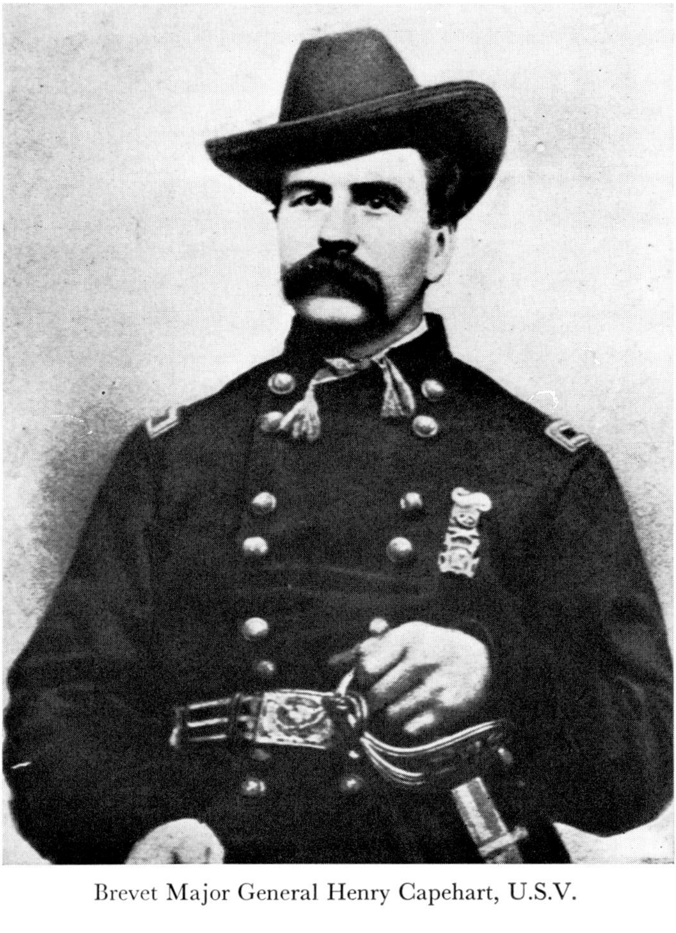

Brevet Major General Henry Capehart, U.S.V.

and he had again married before the war. One daughter survived from this marriage.

Doctor Capehart, an ardent horseman, became the surgeon (rank of major) of the First West Virginia Cavalry on September 6, 1861 (*Heitman*). All of his military experience would be in the cavalry and closely related to this regiment. In 1861, they served in the Army of West Virginia under Generals Rosecrans and Lander. In 1862, they were with Generals Banks and Shields in the Army of the Shenandoah, engaged in the battles at Kernstown and Port Republic. Most of their service, however, was the drudgery of scouting and outpost duty away from the army. In 1863, Capehart was the surgeon-in-chief of the cavalry brigade of General H. E. Davies and of the division of Judson Kilpatrick during the Gettysburg and Bristoe Station campaigns (O.R. 27). General Kilpatrick wrote that he had done his duty like a brave and gallant gentleman, and Davies credited him with having helped to preserve the command.

On December 26, 1863, Surgeon Capehart was made the colonel of the regiment—a most extraordinary vote of confidence. In 1864, they campaigned in the Shenandoah valley under Generals Averell, Crook, Hunter and, finally, Sheridan. Colonel Capehart was assigned a cavalry brigade of four New York and West Virginia regiments in September. The brigade participated under Sheridan in the important battles of Winchester, Fisher's Hill, and Cedar Creek. For this, they were thanked for having labored incessantly without a murmur since May, " . . often barefooted, bareheaded, ragged and lousy from lack of clothing and time to keep themselves clean . . " (*O.R. 28*). Finally they helped Custer to break up Early's army at Waynesborough despite the stiff opposition of Rosser's and other cavalry. Here, Colonel Capehart's brigade reported the capture of 220 prisoners, 300 horses and mules, and three battle flags as well as the destruction of five pieces of artillery, seventy-four wagons of ammunition and stores, two railroad depots, 3,000 rounds of fixed ammunition, 500,000 rounds of rifle ammunition, fifty kegs of powder, 1,500 stand of arms, 500 wall tents, 1,500 cotton quilts, 1,000 pounds of bacon, forty-five hogsheads of tobacco, one tobacco factory and contents, fifteen miles of railroad, 500 kegs of tobacco, 600 5-lb. bales of smoking tobacco, and one canal lock (*O.R. 29*). They then joined Sheridan for the final drive to Appomattox. After the surrender, Sheridan recommended Capehart's promotion to brigadier general for his zeal and energy displayed from Winchester to the James River, for gallantry in the cavalry engagement at Waynesborough, and for distinguished services in the cavalry engagements at Dinwiddie Court House on March 31, 1865, the battles of Five Forks on April 1st and Sailor's Creek on April 6th, and the cavalry engagements at Appomattox Depot and Court House on April 8-9 (*O.R. 29*). Colonel Capehart was finally brevetted a brigadier under date of March 13, 1865 and a major general on June 17, 1865. At the Victory Parade in May, he led his brigade up Pennsylvania avenue. He was mustered out in July. In 1895, just two months before his death, he was awarded the Medal of Honor for having saved under fire the life of a drowning soldier in 1864 (*Heitman*). He was invariably praised highly in the post-combat reports of his superiors, but he wrote no reports, even after he had led a brigade in important battles, and he left virtually no military correspondence in the records. Few of equivalent rank and duty assignments did so little paper work. The omission might have retarded his promotion, and it may indicate modesty.

Doctor Capehart resumed the practice of medicine at Bridgeport, Ohio but his health steadily declined (*Nat. Arch.*). From 1873 to 1881, he lived at Martin's Ferry, Ohio, when he moved to Fargo, North Dakota. This move was made because of backache and vertigo and because he lacked enough strength to practice in the hilly country of eastern Ohio on horseback, so he moved to the level prairie country where he could practice with buggy or phaeton. In Ohio, he had spent much time in bed, and he had tried to supplement his income by drug and local coal businesses, concealing his disabilities from the public. He traced his illness to a severe attack of rheumatism which began on March 31, 1865 at Five Forks, Virginia. It followed a period of severe exposure, and was characterized by stiffness of the joints and soreness in all of his muscles, oppression in the left chest, pain in the back and left hip, and edema enough of the left leg to fill his riding boot. He was never entirely well thereafter. From 1890, he suffered also from palpitation and exertional dyspnea. He died on April 15, 1895, at age seventy, of heart failure attributed to rheumatism contracted in the army. At Fargo, he had served on the pension board.

In summary, this physician, after a successful period as a regimental surgeon in the cavalry, became the colonel of the regiment and, finally, of a brigade. In some of the most difficult and strenuous cavalry service of the war, he won from able superior officers a recommendation for promotion, and he was awarded the brevet grades of brigadier and major general and a Medal of Honor. He had led a brigade for many months without having the corresponding rank. He resumed the practice of medicine, but in the face of deteriorating health from heart disease, allegedly the sequel of an acute rheumatism experienced during his army service and only partly relieved by moving to a level country, he was forced to lead a restricted professional life. He was successful in both of his chosen professions.

9. Brigadier General Robert Francis Catterson, U.S.V.

Robert Catterson was born on a farm in Marion county, Indiana on March 22, 1835 (*Warner*). His father, an Irish immigrant, died when he was five but he obtained an education at Adrian College in Michigan and graduated at a medical school in Cincinnati. He was practicing in Rushville, Indiana in 1861.

Catterson, aged twenty-six, enlisted at once as a private in the Fourteenth Indiana Volunteers. The first colonel of this regiment was Doctor Nathan Kimball, whose biography is also herein presented. Under Kimball, the regiment had service in western Virginia, the Shenandoah Valley, and Maryland. Doctor Catterson was promptly promoted to first sergeant in June, 1861, to second lieutenant in July, and to captain in May, 1862 (*Heitman; Ind. Adj. Gen.*). In this capacity, he was wounded four times in the battle of Antietam. When he was able for duty, he was appointed the lieutenant colonel of the Ninety-seventh Indiana in October, 1862 and its colonel in November (*Indiana Soldiers*). With this regiment, he served in the Army of the Tennessee, usually in its Fifteenth Corps. They went through the campaigns for Vicksburg, Atlanta, Savannah, and the Carolinas. Colonel Catterson led a brigade at Griswoldville, Georgia in November, 1864 and through

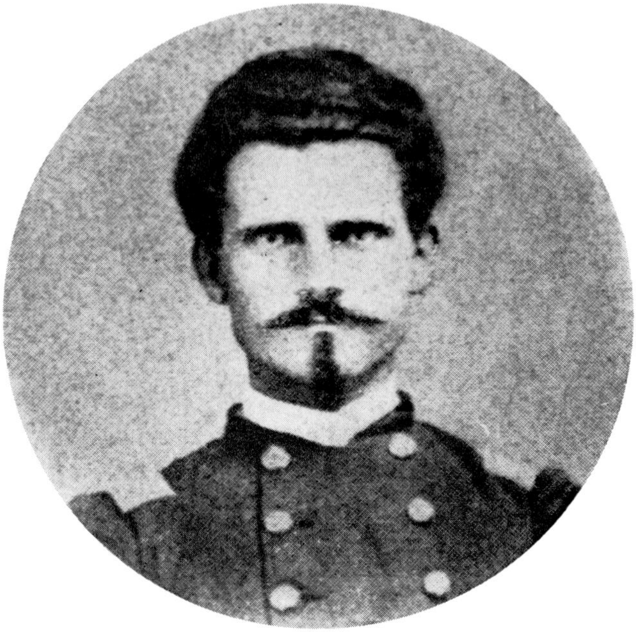

Brigadier General Robert F. Catterson, U.S.V.

the Carolinas in 1865, including the last battle—that at Bentonville. For a short time, he was chief-of-staff to General John Logan of the Fifteenth Corps (*O.R. 30*). He was promoted to brigadier general in the volunteer service on May 31, 1865, and honorably discharged at Louisville on July 26th. He later certified that he had been in forty-one battles and double that number of smaller affairs (*Nat. Arch.*).

Doctor Catterson did not escape unscathed during this time. In January-February, 1864 he was recorded as sick in camp, and from June 25 to August 1, 1864 he was sick in a hospital (*Nat. Arch.; O.R. 31, 32*). The nature of these illnesses has not been found. The Antietam wounds were of greater importance as one of them left permanent effects. A piece of shell struck the right patella but caused little damage. Another shell fragment or a musket ball cut across the base of the left thumb. Another ball entered the outer side of the left foot, struck the bones and, passing backward, lodged under the integuments beneath the middle of the os calcis, from where it was extracted. Finally, a ball entered the right gluteus muscle just posterior to the rim of the right acetabulum, passed backward, and made its exit at the posterior part of the lacerated sphincter ani; it then passed through a part of the left gluteal muscle. He was taken first to the hospital of the Third Division, Second Corps. From there, he was moved on September 24th to the Second General Hospital at Frederick and on the 26th to the Seminary General Hospital at Georgetown (*Nat. Arch.*). His subsequent statement that his wounds were first dressed (because of the great number of wounded) at the Seminary Hospital eleven days after the battle seems hardly credible. In 1900, the pension board at Sauk Center, Minnesota found that the rectal wound had been three or four inches up and that, on healing, a pouch or sacculation persisted that sometimes filled with a mass of coagulated blood that interfered with defecation. The threat of postoperative infection still discouraged attempts at surgical repair at that time.

Doctor Catterson did not return to medicine. Instead, he first became a cotton speculator and carpet-bagger politician in Arkansas (*Warner*). He was variously the U. S. Marshal, Mayor of Little Rock, and commander of Negro militia. After reconstruction, he lived in Chicago, Minneapolis, and Sauk Center, but he was not very successful in business or farming. He died in San Antonio, Texas on March 30, 1914 after a stroke, and was buried there in the National Cemetery. As he was seventy-nine years old, the persistent war injury had not appreciably shortened his life.

In summary, this physician went from private to colonel in nineteen months and to brigadier general by the end of the war, when he had already performed the duties of this grade for about four months. Four times wounded in one battle, he carried disability to the grave. He did not resume medical practice, and was not very successful as politician, farmer, or business man.

10. Brevet Brigadier General Thomas E. Champion, U.S.V.

Thomas E. Champion was born at Palmyra, New York on August 3, 1825 (*Eddy; Nat. Arch.; Partridge*). At the age of twelve, he was taken to Michigan where he worked on a farm for four years.

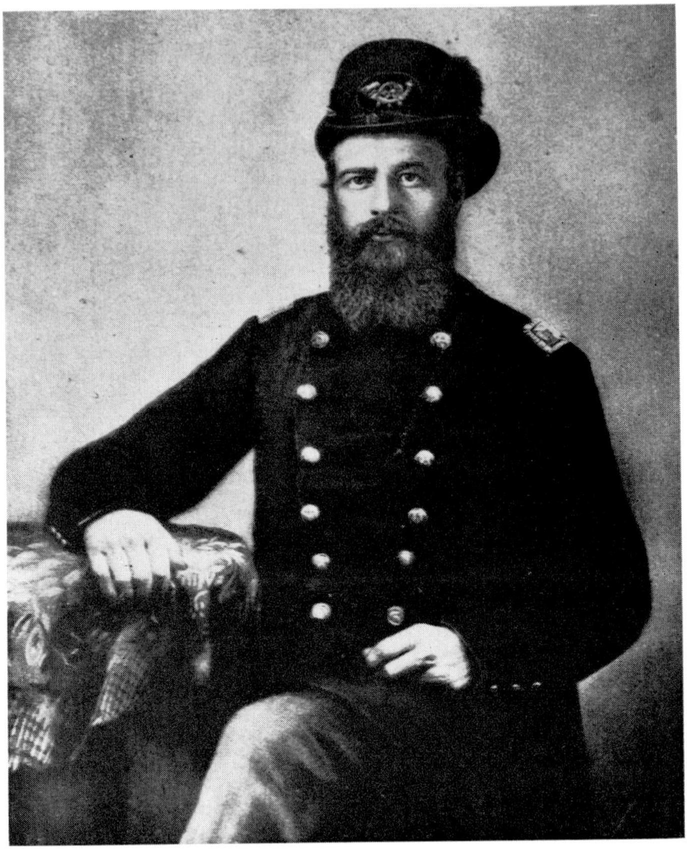

Brevet Brigadier General Thomas E. Champion, U.S.V.

He was then employed in a printing office while studying medicine in his leisure time. He graduated from the University of Michigan and was admitted to medical practice in 1847. He was married the following year, and he moved to Freeport, Illinois in 1850 and to Warren in 1851, where he practiced medicine. In the meantime, he studied law and was admitted to the bar in 1856. His legal practice was soon large. He was a distinguished speaker and a robust man of commanding appearance with a powerful voice.

In 1862, Champion raised a company, which became a part of the Ninety-sixth Illinois Volunteers. In camp at Rockford, he was elected the captain of the company and then the colonel of the regiment, although he had no military training. However, he studied the manuals and became a good drillmaster. The first winter was spent in the Department of the Ohio, on guard duty at various places in Kentucky and Tennessee. The men suffered severely from the camp diseases. In passing through Harrodsburg, Kentucky, for example, they left behind fifty men sick mostly with measles. In camp at Danville, so many were sick, including the surgeon and the second assistant surgeon, that a company captain—a physician—was detailed to assist the first assistant surgeon (*Partridge*). Former lawyer Champion protected his men from lawsuits that followed foraging and occasionally he addressed them but as an ex-physician he did not keep them healthy.

The regiment joined the Army of the Cumberland of Rosecrans for the summer campaign toward Chattanooga in 1863. Their initial battle came at Chickamauga in September. The regiment entered the fight with 401 officers and men and it had 225 casualties (*O.R. 33*). This was the price they paid to help General George Thomas win his "Rock" sobriquet. The colonel and his men were especially commended for bold impetuosity, efficiency, and gallantry. Champion had two horses shot under him, his clothes were pierced, and he himself fired a musket for a time. The regiment fought again at Lookout Mountain, in Sherman's Atlanta Campaign of 1864, and with Thomas against Hood at Nashville that December. Its total deaths eventually numbered 219, of whom 112 died of combat wounds and 107 of disease. In addition, many hundreds had been wounded or sick. Despite the medical degree of its colonel, the regiment, for example, suffered severely from scurvy in the winter camp of 1863-64, and at one time in April, 1864 there were fifty well-defined cases; they had swollen sore gums with loose teeth, swollen painful limbs, languor, and depression. Vegetables—generally potatoes and sour kraut—were obtained when possible.

Colonel Champion was first assigned to the command of a brigade of four regiments in July, 1863 (*O.R. 34*). From this time, he alternated between regimental and brigade commands. However, his health deteriorated steadily beginning in December, 1862, so that nearly half the time thereafter was spent on sick leaves at home in Illinois or in military hospitals. Moreover, Colonel Champion was severely wounded in the face by a bullet in June, 1864 near Kenesaw Mountain (*Partridge; O.R. 35*). Bone was painfully injured, his general condition was poor, and the wound healed slowly. When he rejoined at the end of September, the wound had closed, but his health was still bad and in appearance he had aged many years since June. Already at the time of the examination for his first sick leave, in April of 1863, the surgeon found infraclavicular deformity of the right chest, bilateral areas of consolidation in several lobes, constant moist crepitations, and irritation of the entire bronchial tract in a person having a hereditary tuberculous diathesis (*Nat. Arch.*). Eight months later a severe cough, mucopurulent expectorations, bronchitis, pain in the side, and an increase in the areas of consolidation were recorded. A board of examiners at Lookout Mountain in November, 1864 found him suffering from a severe contusion of the perineum and testicle, producing orchitis, prostatitis, and hydrocele, the consequence of an injury received in September. It is possible if not probable that these lesions were tuberculous.

Colonel Champion never returned to active duty and he was never again well. He had been recommended for promotion but the lists were full. He was, however, awarded the rank of brevet brigadier general to date from February 20, 1865, and he resigned on June 7th of that year. He settled in Knoxville, Tennessee for his health, and resumed the practice of law. But he was not well and considered going to California for his "lungs." However, he died of consumption on June 13, 1873, aged forty-seven, leaving a wife, three sons and a daughter.

In summary, this physician, after nine years of practice, abandoned medicine in favor of law. Although he had no prior military training, he became the colonel of a regiment and eventually of a brigade of eight regiments. He was successful in this third profession despite a steady decline in physical condition from tuberculosis. He was twice wounded in battle, and was finally awarded the grade of brigadier general by brevet. There is no evidence in his military record that he had a medical education. He died from the progression of his tuberculosis eight years after the war. The assignment of an infantry captain in his regiment, who was also a physician, to temporary medical duty during a period of need was not unusual in that war.

11. Brevet Major General Samuel Wylie Crawford, U.S.A.

Samuel W. Crawford was the army doctor in Fort Sumter when it fell. He soon transferred to the infantry, rose to a divisional command in the volunteer service, remained in the regular army after the war, and after 1861 evinced no interest in medicine. He was born near Chambersburg, Pennsylvania on November 8, 1827 (*Hume*). His father, the Reverend Dr. Samuel W. Crawford, became the Principal of the Academy of the University of Pennsylvania three years later, and he died before the war (*Crawford*). The Samuel of this sketch was awarded by the University the degrees of B.A. in 1846, M.A. in 1849, M.D. in 1850, and an honorary LL.D. in 1867. His doctoral thesis on *Hypertrophy and Atrophy*

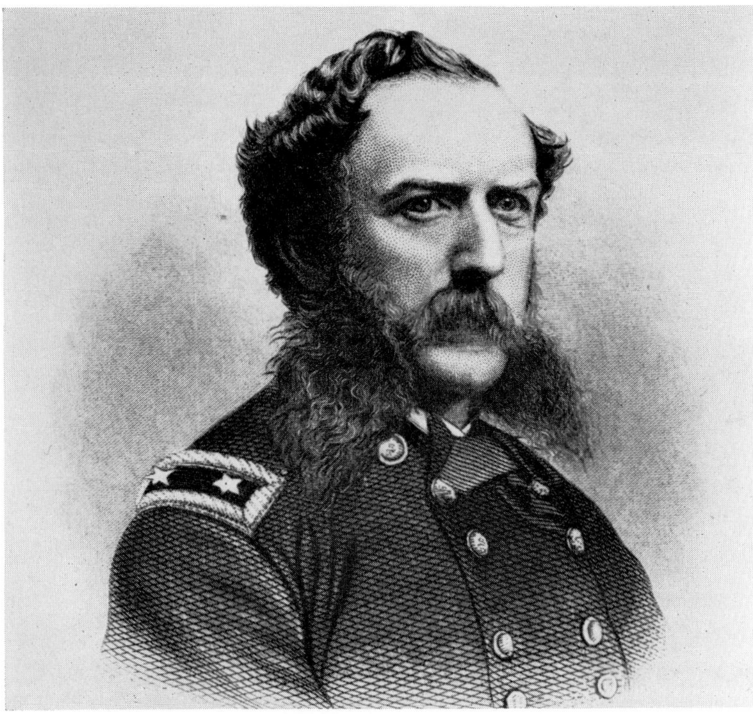

Brevet Major General Samuel W. Crawford, U.S.A.

was a good textbook discussion of these phenomena but it contributed nothing new (*Crawford, 1850*). The honorary degree was awarded " . . on account of his eminent learning." Crawford's scholarly book on *The Genesis of the Civil War* was published only in 1887 (*Crawford*), and no grounds have been found for the citation of 1867.

Doctor Crawford became an assistant surgeon in the army in 1851. During the next ten years he had a wide variety of assignments at forts and on expeditions in the Western territories and in Mexico, in exploration or Indian fighting. He simultaneously served as a naturalist, collecting specimens of birds for Baird of the Smithsonian Institution. In September, 1860, he was ordered to the forts in Charleston Harbor to succeed a surgeon dead supposedly of yellow fever. He changed the diagnosis of the epidemic to dengue fever, and there was no further mortality. During the following months, he won the confidence of Major Robert Anderson, serving as a military advisor, acting quartermaster and commissary, senior watch officer, and meteorologist as well as post surgeon. He also sold sketches to *Harper's Weekly* and kept notes for his later historical writing. His own health was impaired by a bad throat. During the bombardment of the fort he voluntarily acted as a battery commander. In politics he was a unionist but not an abolitionist.

Back in the North, Surgeon Crawford was commissioned a major in the Thirteenth Infantry. During the first winter, he was an aide on the staff of General Rosecrans in West Virginia. In April, 1862, he was suddenly promoted to brigadier general of volunteers and placed in the command of an infantry brigade in what soon became Pope's Army of Virginia. At the end of the Second Bull Run Campaign in August, he came into the Army of the Potomac, in which he served until Appomattox. With this army he went through some of the heaviest fighting of the war, assigned variously as a brigade, divisional, and temporary corps commander, of the Fifth Corps.

General Crawford was wounded at the battle of Antietam and injured at the battle of Spotsylvania Court House. While leading a division at Antietam on September 17, 1862, he suffered a gunshot wound in the thigh. As was customary, he retained the command until he was exhausted by the loss of blood (*O.R. 36*). He was out of the field for five months, but he had court duty in Washington during a part of this time. At Spotsylvania on May 8, 1864, he was injured by a blow from a falling tree limb cut off by a cannon ball, but he relinquished his divisional command only for a few hours.

After the war, General Crawford reverted to his regular rank of lieutenant colonel, but he became the colonel of the Sixteenth Infantry in 1869. He also was promoted by brevets in the regular army to brigadier and major general. In 1873, he retired for disability. The Antietam gunshot wound, nine years old, had broken down and was giving off constant and exhausting discharges (*Nat. Arch.*). In 1875, he was awarded the rank of brigadier in the regular army by a special act of Congress (*Heitman*).

Crawford lived for nineteen years longer, dying suddenly in 1892 at age sixty-four. During this time he wrote his history of the coming of the war. He traveled extensively in Europe and took an interest in historical and geographical societies. His health at times was not good because of poorly documented illnesses, and it is known that he consulted Charcot in Paris at least once (*Crawford papers*). Among the causes of the invalidism and death to be considered must be included the possible late complications of chronic osteomyelitis such as an amyloid nephrosis.

An injustice has been done to Crawford in history consequent to his Antietam wound. It has been suggested in a number of places that he exaggerated its effects for personal advantage. The wound was thought to have involved only the soft tissues of the thigh so that it should have healed promptly, yet he was out for five months. From its behavior in 1873, however, it is now known that the femur had been injured and that necrosis followed. As the result of vascular injury or infection, introduced then or later, the end result was a chronic osteomyelitis. Occurring as it did in a major weight-bearing bone, it was important. In the absence of roentgenograms or surgical exploration under direct vision, the correct diagnosis could not have been made sooner than it was, but the imputations that he was a malingerer are unfair.

Crawford appears to have been moderately competent as an infantry general. He did not inspire his men and was not popular with his superiors. The justification for his promotion to general grade at a time when he had little or no experience is not apparent. It is known that he used political influence to gain personal advantage although this would not have been necessary.

Nothing in Crawford's record after Fort Sumter suggests that he had a medical education and had practiced military medicine for ten years. His troops were not healthier nor cared for better in battle or in camp than were others. His vast exposure over a period of twenty years to the problems of hygiene, sanitation, and epidemiology among troops under varying conditions led to no new medical knowledge. His transfer from medicine to the infantry appears to have been motivated by the possibility of greater distinction and by a weak interest in medicine. Possibly, his most important legacy was his book on the genesis of the war. His considerable talents in administration were needed by the medical department, and one wonders about his fate if he had remained a surgeon.

12. Brevet Brigadier General Daniel Dustin, U.S.V.

Daniel Dustin was born on October 5, 1820 in Topsham, Vermont. He spent his boyhood there, and graduated in medicine from Dartmouth College in 1846 (*Dustin*). Until 1858, he practiced in Vermont and in California, and thereafter in Sycamore, Illinois. In 1855 and 1856, he represented Nevada County in the California legislature.

Doctor Dustin became the captain of Company I, Eighth Illinois Cavalry in September, 1861 and a major in the following January. This regiment was assembled at St. Charles, Illinois. The contract for their food was $0.16 daily per man whereas their horses were fed for only $0.14 (*Hard*). This was one of the few "Western" regiments in the Army of the Potomac. Although the surgeons were overworked by a sick list of over five hundred men (mostly typhoid and typho-malarial fever) in January, and an epidemic of measles in February, Major Dustin did not help them as a physician. He resigned in September, 1862 at the end of McClellan's Peninsular campaign to become the colonel of the One Hundred and Fifth Illinois Infantry, a regiment then being recruited (*Nat. Arch.*).

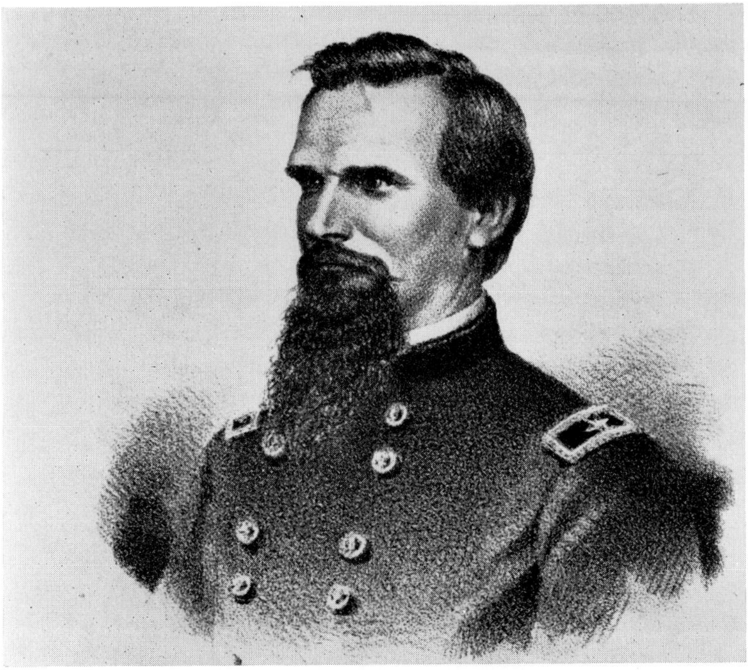

Brevet Brigadier General Daniel Dustin, U.S.V.

This regiment had guard and garrison duty at various places in Kentucky and Tennessee until April, 1864, when it was brigaded in the Third Division, Twentieth corps, Army of the Cumberland (General George Thomas). With this corps they went to Atlanta, Savannah, and Washington under Sherman. From August, 1864, Dustin was in brigade command except during short leaves of absence or while he temporarily led the division of fifteen regiments (*O.R. 37*). Colonel Benjamin Harrison (later President) had the Seventieth Indiana in Dustin's brigade. Dustin was promoted to brigadier general by brevet on March 16, 1865 for gallant services in Georgia and South Carolina, and he was mustered out in June. The only recorded illness in service was an attack of diarrhea in August, 1862 that required a sick leave. Dustin's official post-action reports reveal strenuous soldiering (*O.R. Index*).

Doctor Dustin returned to the practice of medicine in Sycamore, but his political interests soon returned and dominated. He was elected the clerk of DeKalb County in the Fall of 1865 and, later, the county treasurer. Then followed the clerkship of the circuit court, a position he held for ten years. In addition, he was a trustee of the Soldier's and Sailor's Home at Quincy. By appointment, he became the U.S. Assistant Treasurer at Chicago in 1890. His first wife died in 1850 and he remarried four years later (*Nat. Arch.*). He died on March 30, 1892 of "paralysis," leaving a widow and four children.

In summary, this is another example of an eastern-born physician who took Greely's advice but eventually wound up in Illinois. He dabbled in politics as a side line both before and after the war. In his three professions—medicine, politics, and military—he seemed relatively most distinguished if not competent in the third. It appears that his interest in medicine was weak.

13. Brevet Brigadier General Samuel McKenzie Elliott, U.S.V.

Samuel Elliott was born at Inverness, Scotland on April 9, 1811. He graduated at the College of Surgeons, Glasgow, in 1828, and carried out research on the anatomy and the effects of climate on the eye (*C.A.B.*). In 1833, he migrated to the United States, where he continued medical studies in Cincinnati and Philadelphia. He began a practice limited to diseases of the eye in New York City in 1835. Successful from the start, he was, however, considered irregular and unprofessional for keeping discoveries secret. He therefore obtained a diploma after an examination in the "New York Medical College," and gave lectures explaining his methods. Eccentric and successful, he was described as amiable, generous to charities, and friendly.

Doctor Elliott organized the Seventy-ninth New York Infantry Regiment, which was mustered in on May 29, 1861 with himself as the lieutenant colonel (*Heitman; Phisterer; Todd*). Known also as the Cameron Rifle Highlanders, Highland Guard, and by other names, they departed New York without training on June 2nd for the front near Washington. Here, they were eventually joined by their colonel, J. C. Cameron, a brother of the Secretary of War. The regiment had about 800 men exclusive of the band and drum

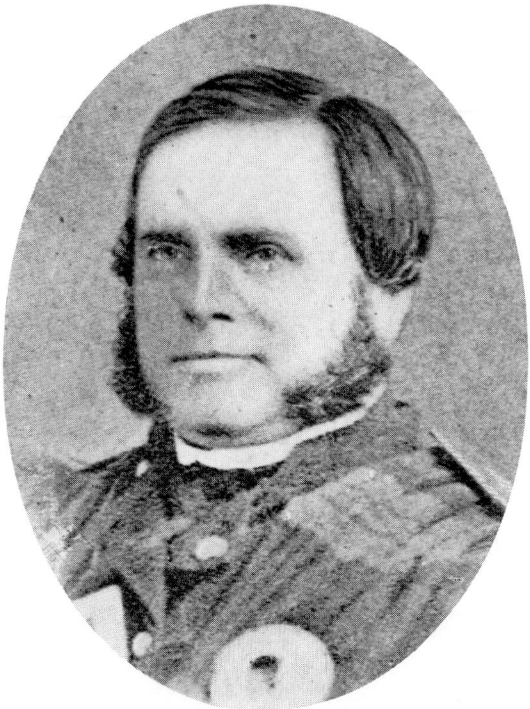

Brevet Brigadier General Samuel Elliott, U.S.V.

corps; among them were three sons of Doctor Elliott (*Moore*). Colonel Cameron was killed at First Bull Run among the 198 casualties of the regiment (*Sherman*), and Lieutenant Colonel Elliott was left in the command until Colonel Isaac Stevens arrived to take over. On August 14th, most of the regiment refused to obey the orders of the new colonel in a mix-up of conflicting instructions issued by the state and federal authorities (*Stevens; Todd*). General McClellan published a scathing denunciation. As a consequence, the lieutenant colonel was required to resign his commission, and he had no further service in the war. Nevertheless, he was later awarded the rank of brevet brigadier general to date from March 13, 1865. He was appointed the colonel of another regiment in October, 1861 and of the Seventy-ninth in 1864, but was not mustered in for either position and, as far as is known did not serve. The promotion must have acquitted him of any wrong in the affair in August.

According to one account, Lieutenant Colonel Elliott's horse was shot in battle at First Bull Run, falling on him and injuring his spine so that he was disabled for further active service (*C.A.B.*). The historian of the regiment, in contrast, claims he was absent from this battle *(Todd)*. There is no pension file or military service record on this officer, and the published *Official Records* are uniquely silent on him.

Doctor Elliott resumed practice until 1874, when he retired to his residence on Staten Island. Here, he died on April 30, 1875 of "disease of the heart" (*Elliott*). His war record shows good intentions if not military competence. It is peculiarly difficult in retrospect to judge both his medical and his military careers.

14. Brevet Brigadier General John Johnson Elwell, U.S.V.

John J. Elwell was born on a farm near Warren, Ohio on June 22, 1820 (*DAB; Reid; Shastid*). He was educated in the schools of Warren and at Western Reserve University. He graduated as a Doctor of Medicine at the Cleveland Medical College in 1846 and practiced at Orwell, Ohio for nine years. In 1853-54, he represented Ashtabula County in the Ohio legislature. In 1854, he was admitted to the bar and thereafter he practiced law in Cleveland, specializing in legal medicine. He also lectured on medical jurisprudence at Ohio State University, and the Union Law College. In 1857, he established as editor and publisher the *Western Law Monthly*. In 1860, he published his book on *Medical Jurisprudence: A Medico-Legal Treatise on Malpractice and Medical Evidence* (*Elwell*). This book, the first treatise in English on the subject, was clear, comprehensive, and timely. It became an authority in the United States, Canada, and Great Britain, eventually passing through four editions.

Doctor Elwell entered the army on August 3, 1861 as an assistant quartermaster with the rank of captain in the volunteer service. In 1862, he was an aide to General Henry W. Benham at Secessionville, South Carolina (*O.R. 38*), and on the staff of General O. M. Mitchell at Hilton Head (*O.R. 39*). In 1863, he became the chief

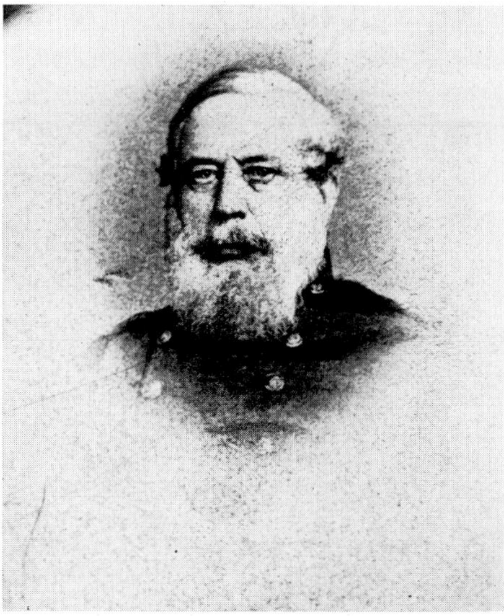

Brevet Brigadier General John J. Elwell, U.S.V.

quartermaster of the Tenth Army Corps and of the Department of the South with the temporary rank of lieutenant colonel, serving successively under Generals David Hunter and Q. A. Gillmore (*Nat. Arch.; O.R. 40, 41*). In February, 1864, because of reduced health, he was assigned to quartermaster duty at the draft rendezvous and the prison camp at Elmira, New York, reverting to the rank of captain. At the end of the war, he was among those especially cited by the quartermaster department for faithful and meritorious service (*O.R. 42*), so he was eventually awarded the grade of brevet brigadier general of volunteers to date from March 13, 1865. He was mustered out on March 16, 1866 (*Heitman*).

Lieutenant Colonel Elwell was handicapped by bad health and misfortune. He was stricked with yellow fever at Port Royal, South Carolina in 1863 (*Shastid*). Also, in March of that year, his right leg was badly fractured below the knee when his horse fell through a bridge upon him (*Nat. Arch.*). The fracture was oblique in both bones and the joint cartilages were injured. He was left with a partial ankylosis, three quarters of an inch of shortening of the leg, and impaired motion. In October, 1864, at Elmira the leg was again fractured when a frightened team threw him violently upon some stones. The femoral condyles were fractured and the old joint injury exacerbated. Six weeks later, while he was descending a stairway on crutches, he fell to the bottom and obliquely fractured the same femur in its lower third and further injured the joint. The end result was nearly two inches of shortening, a crooked leg, atrophied muscles, and a weak knee with an impaired range of motion. He was never again entirely strong and he moved with a decided limp.

Because of total and permanent disability, Elwell was granted a pension of $30.00 per month. In 1875, the award was reduced to $20.00, and the higher amount was never restored despite repeated applications.

Elwell returned to the practice of law, teaching, and writing in law and medicine. He contributed to and edited *Bouvier's Law Dictionary,* wrote for the scholarly *North American Review,* published on the sanity of Guiteau, the assassin of President Garfield, and revised his book on medical jurisprudence. His wife and four children having died, he adopted the three children of a brother, leaving them his fortune. He was Professor of Medical Jurisprudence at Western Reserve from 1865-1872 (*Waite*). He died on March 13, 1900, aged seventy-nine years.

In summary, after nine years of practice this physician turned to law, specializing in legal medicine. For reasons that have not been revealed, he served during the war as a quartermaster instead of in the medical or legal departments. Left a partial cripple by service-incurred injuries, he nevertheless had a full and successful career in the legal, educational, and related fields.

15. Brigadier General Richard Montgomery Gano, C.S.A.

Richard Gano was born in Bourbon County, Kentucky on June 17, 1830 (*Evans; Warner*). His father was a minister and stockman (*Gano, 1952*). He attended Bacon College at Harrodsburg, Kentucky, Bethany College in Virginia, and the University of Louisville, where he graduated in medicine in 1850 (*Gano, 1913*). He practiced medicine in Bourbon County for eight years and in Tarrant County, Texas until the war. In 1860-61, he was a member of the Texas legislature. There is no record of any military training, although he served on the frontier during Indian warfare.

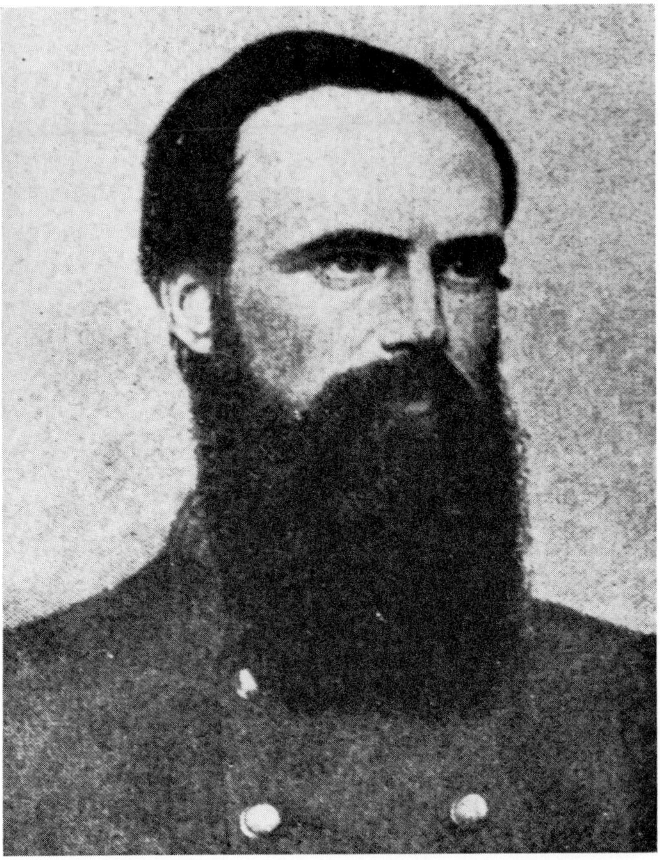

Brigadier General Richard M. Gano, C.S.A.

In 1861, Captain Gano recruited "Gano's Squadron" of two Texas companies for service with General A. S. Johnston. After Johnston's death, he led the Seventh Kentucky Cavalry of Morgan's Cavalry, raiding into Kentucky from bases in Tennessee. He led successively a squadron, battalion, and regiment, meanwhile advancing from captain to colonel (*O.R. Index*). In April, 1863, Colonel Gano attempted to resign because of poor health (*Nat. Arch.*), but he was ordered to the Trans-Mississippi Department of General E. Kirby Smith. Here, he was placed in charge of all Texas State Cavalry (*O.R. 43*). Later, he led the Texas Brigade in the Indian Territory and Arkansas (*O.R. 44*). In 1864, he contended with several Union generals, also physicians (Blunt, Kimball), although this fact was probably unknown to them all. The service out here was not attractive and desertions became numerous (*O.R. 45, 46*). In the battle at Jenkin's Ferry, Arkansas against Steele in April, he was wounded (*O.R. 47*). Although he had held the command of a brigade for over a year, and had repeatedly been recommended for promotion to general, he was not appointed to this rank until March, 1865.

The illness of 1863 was diagnosed valvular disease and hypertrophy of the heart by several physicians, including D. Y. Yandell, his old teacher and now surgeon and the medical director of Hardee's Corps (*Nat. Arch.*). He was pronounced unfit for active service and in need of quiet and rest to prolong his life. In January, 1864, he was on sick leave (*O.R. 48*). The wound in April was a flesh wound of the arm that left some permanent disability.

In 1866, Gano became a minister and evangelist in the Christian church. He was also a stockman, an officer and stockholder in banks and large business enterprises in Texas, and active in the United Confederate Veteran's Association. He died at the home of a daughter in Dallas on March 27, 1913, of senile debility, aged eighty-two years. If he had organic heart disease in 1863, it had not shortened his life.

In summary, this subject was successively physician, cavalryman, stockman, and clergyman. He seemed most successful in the latter capacity. Politics and business also took some of his attention. In the war, his service was heavy but, like that of thousands of others, not outstanding, and he participated in no major battle.

16. Brevet Major General Thomas Maley Harris, U.S.V.

Thomas M. Harris was born in rural western Virginia (now Ritchie County, West Virginia) on June 17, 1813 (*C.A.B.; Lang; Matheny*). He attended school for three months in a log cabin in 1823 and Marietta College briefly, but he was largely self-educated. Nevertheless, he taught in rural schools in Ohio and at the Parkersburg Institute. During these years, he was also studying medicine with the local practitioners. He graduated in medicine in 1843 at the University of Louisville after one term of study and returned home to practice. Eventually, he accumulated large tracts of unim-

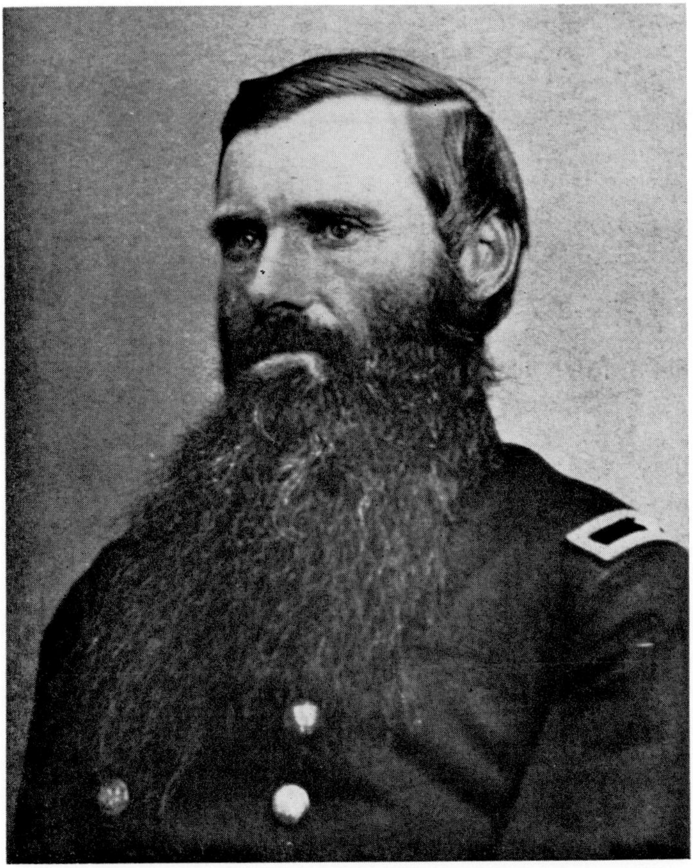

Brevet Major General Thomas M. Harris, U.S.V.

proved land, some of it for oil speculation. In 1841, he married a school teacher. They had four children, one of whom died in infancy. In politics, Doctor Harris had been an old line Whig and, in the crisis, he became a strong Unionist. He published a religious tract on *Calvinism Vindicate*d in 1860.

Harris was practicing medicine at Glenville, Gilmer County, Virginia when the war began. He started recruiting what became the Tenth West Virginia Infantry Volunteers in August, 1861. Although he was widely known, recruitment proved difficult in this divided country, and the regiment was not filled until 1862. As the companies were filled, they were set to work patrolling to suppress partisans and bushwhackers. Doctor Harris became the lieutenant colonel of the regiment in March and its colonel on May 20th of that year. He was familiar with the mountains and roads and was assigned to the patrol of a large area successively by departmental commanders Generals John Fremont (*O.R. 49*), John Wool (*O.R. 50*), B. F. Kelley (*O.R. 50*), Robert C. Schenck (*O.R. 51*), W. W. Averell (*O.R. 52*), Franz Sigel (*O.R. 53*), and others. For nearly three years, Colonel Harris' duty was much like that of Colonel Capehart (see case 8) but even more strenuous; much of it dealt essentially with the control of guerilla activity and guarding the Baltimore and Ohio Railroad. Finally, in 1864, this regiment, now assigned to a brigade which Colonel Harris commanded, came into the main stream of the war in the Shenandoah Valley Campaign of Generals George Crook and Phil Sheridan. The casualties in the small brigade of Colonel Harris became heavier—for example, 238 at the battle of Winchester, 41 at Fisher's Hill, 176 at Cedar Creek, and 209 at Strasburg (*O.R. 54*). Of Fisher's Hill, Colonel Harris wrote in his report that . . "During the greater portion of this time I was engaged in urging forward the more timid and weak, and driving from cover the cowardly, . ." (*O.R. 55*). At the urging of the Wheeling government, he was promoted to brigadier general by brevet in December, to date from October 19, 1864. After Early's army had been soundly defeated, Harris, now leading a division, was shipped to City Point, where he came into the Twenty-fourth Corps of General John Gibbon in the Army of the James for the final campaign of 1865. On April 2nd, his brigade, to the command of which he had reverted, assaulted and carried Fort Baldwin in the Petersburg line. On April 9th, the brigade was in the front line at Appomattox and about to charge when the hostilities were announced ended (*O.R. 56*). Although Harris had repeatedly been recommended for promotion and had for brief periods led a division—a command calling for a major general—he was not made a full brigadier until March 29, 1865. Later, he was brevetted a major general to date from April 2nd for his gallant conduct in the assault on Petersburg (*Heitman*). He had aroused much ill will in his brigade for his stern discipline, but he was regarded as able.

General Harris was appointed by President Johnson in 1865 to membership on the military commission to try the Lincoln conspirators. Among other things, they found the Confederate government not involved, although Harris was not certain. It is said that Mrs. Surratt was hung chiefly because of the influence of Generals Harris and Lew Wallace (*Matheny*). The qualifications of Doctor Harris for this important position were not stated. He knew no law and had little political influence. He came from a border area. Presumably he was selected for sensible and sound judgment. He was finally mustered out on April 30, 1866 after having served briefly in the Freedman's Bureau and having declined, on account of his age and poor health, the proffer of a lieutenant colonelcy in the regular army. This unusual offer in itself proves his military competence. From his record, Harris seems to have made a slow start but a strong finish. This was explained by the nature of his assignments; there was no opportunity for distinction in patrolling the valleys of West Virginia.

Doctor Harris resumed the practice of medicine but his health was poor and he gave it up in 1882. He was then occupied principally in farming and politics until invalidism put a stop to them in about 1890. He was elected to the West Virginia legislature in 1867, was adjutant general of the state in 1869-70, and the Federal pension agent at Wheeling from 1871-77. Although he was a Presbyterian, he occasionally preached in the local Methodist church.

Doctor Harris dated a severe and permanent rheumatism to his accidental submersion in ice water in December, 1864, when he was disembarking his command at City Point (*Nat. Arch.*). His fingers and other joints became enlarged and deformed. Painful and sometimes disabling hemorrhoids, present before the war but grown worse during service, were finally cured by the injection into them of carbolic acid in 1883. For his various ailments, he wrote that he had dieted carefully and taken several preparations of pepsin for indigestion; he had used Tr. gent. Comp. and Tr. cinchona Comp. as a heart stimulant; as a nerve tonic and cholegogue he had taken Tr. nux. v. and acid nitro prusiaticum; for rheumatism he had " . . gone over the whole round of rheumatic remidies";

for gout he had taken Succus Alterans, Syr. Sarsap. with potassae iodidi and corrosive sublimate, etc.

Doctor Harris' first wife died in 1885 and he was remarried in 1888. He was nearly blind and deaf when he died in Harrisville, West Virginia on September 30, 1906 at age ninety-three. The cause of death was recorded as disease of the heart. One of his most important contributions was a book on the *Assassination of Lincoln,* published in 1892. He wrote it twenty-seven years after the trial because a new generation had been subjected to an attempt to show that Mrs. Surrett was innocent (*Harris*). Like his voluminous military correspondence published in the *Official Records,* this writing is lucid, orderly and convincing. In the post-war years, he also wrote religious tracts and one implicating the Catholic Church in the Lincoln conspiracy (*Matheny*).

In summary, this general practitioner without known prior military education went directly into the army as a lieutenant colonel of a regiment which he had helped to recruit. He led an infantry brigade and, for a time, a division in some of the heaviest fighting of the war. He was awarded the rank of major general by brevet in the volunteers and served on the commission that tried Lincoln's assassins. Because of declining health, attributed to exposure in the army, he returned only briefly to the practice of medicine, but he performed possibly his greatest public service by writing a book on the assassination of Lincoln. As a preacher, teacher, farmer, physician, soldier, politician and author, Doctor Harris led a full and active life in which medicine was a minor interest.

17. Brevet Brigadier General David Burke Hillis, U.S.V.

David Hillis was born in Jefferson County, Indiana on July 24, 1825 (*Atkinson; Stuart*). His father was a prominent pioneer and politician. He attended South Hanover College in Indiana. During the war with Mexico, he was a private for nine months at New Albany, Indiana. Three months of this time were spent in a hospital on account of measles (*Nat. Arch.*). In 1847, at age twenty-one, he began to practice medicine, first at Rockford, Indiana and then at Brownstown. Three different statements are found on his medical education. According to one he was awarded the M.D. de-

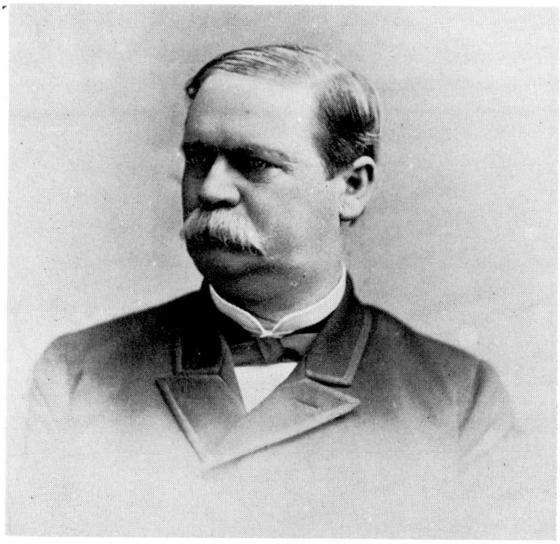

Brevet Brigadier General David Hillis, U.S.V

gree by Washington University, St. Louis (*Hillis*); according to another, he was graduated from the St. Louis Medical College in 1847 and in 1877 (*Atkinson*); according to a third version, he studied medicine at Madison, Indiana in 1846 or 1847 (*Stuart*). This period would coincide with his hospital experience as a soldier and patient in the Mexican War.

In 1858, Doctor Hillis moved to Bloomfield, Iowa and in 1860 to Keokuk. Here he practiced medicine (*Atkinson*) or was in the dry-goods business (*Stuart*), or both.

From August, 1861 to March, 1862, Hillis was an aide to Governor Kirkwood, like Doctor Bussey (see case 6). He then became the lieutenant colonel of the Seventeenth Iowa Infantry and on September 4th the colonel of the regiment (*Heitman*). This outfit was shipped to the front in May after Shiloh without training or proper equipment (*Ingersoll*). It did poorly at the battles of Iuka and Second Corinth under Rosecrans, but eventually it fought well in the Vicksburg Campaign of Grant. Colonel Hillis was commended for distinguished services at the battles of Jackson and Champion Hill in May, prior to the investment (*O.R. 57*). He resigned on May 30, 1863, five weeks before the surrender, and took no further part in the war. Nevertheless, he was awarded the rank of brigadier general by brevet to date from March 13, 1865 (the "Bloody Thirteenth") for meritorious service. Since August, 1862, he had been suffering from attacks of rheumatism involving chiefly the left leg and hip, for which he had taken leave of absence several times (*Nat. Arch.*). He was described as popular and as able to make " . . a pretty forcible extempore speech" (*Stuart*).

Doctor Hillis returned to the practice of medicine at Keokuk, eventually specializing in the diseases of women and children. He was the President of the Board of Health for four years and the health officer of the city. In 1872 he was elected to but declined the chair of obstetric medicine and diseases of women in the Keokuk College of Physicians and Surgeons, but he was the president of this school from 1890 to 1899 (*Hillis*). In 1877, he was a member of the board of visitors to the U. S. Military Academy by appointment of the president. He held membership in the county, state, and national medical societies. He was married in 1848 and again in 1885, two sons surviving from the first marriage. Doctor Hillis died at Keokuk on September 9, 1900 at age seventy-five of apoplexy. For several years, he had received a pension for disability incurred in service and diagnosed as rheumatism with resulting disease of the heart. In 1876, he had suffered a severe attack of acute articular rheumatism involving various joints, complicated by carditis, from which recovery had been slow and incomplete.

In summary, this physician, with no prior military training except that of a private in the Mexican War and an aide to a governor, became a colonel of infantry and had a creditable record until this career was stopped by a service-incurred disease. He resumed the practice of medicine, at which he was successful in several capacities. His death resulted from the late effects of a service-related disease, illustrating again the fact that the war records show only a part of the mortality and morbidity.

18. Brigadier General James Lawlor Kiernan, U.S.V.

James Kiernan was born in Ireland on October 26, 1837. He attended Trinity College, Dublin, and graduated from the medical department of the University of the City of New York in 1857

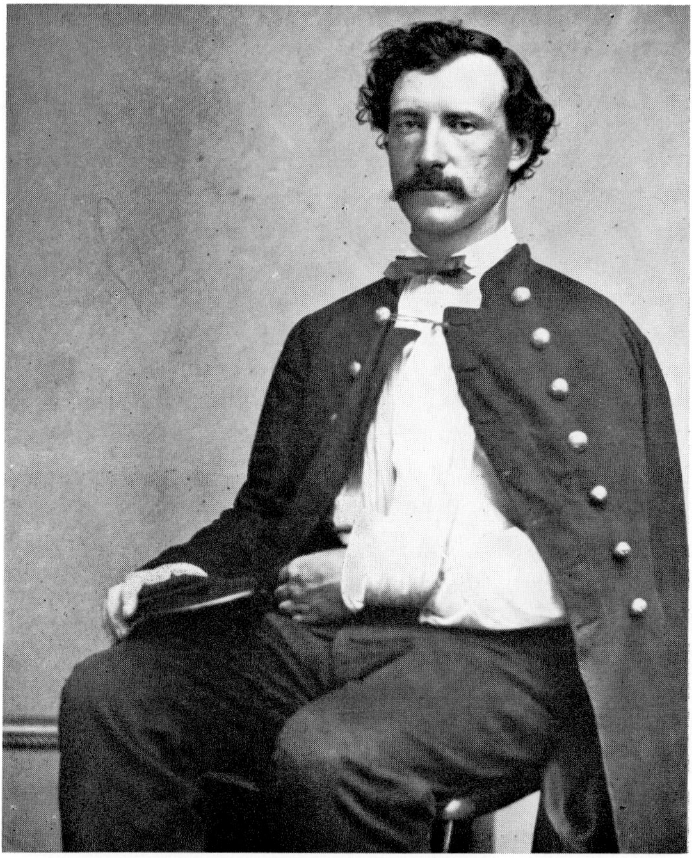

Brigadier General James L. Kiernan, U.S.V.

(*C.A.B.; Warner*). From 1859 to 1861, he practiced with a brother-in-law and was a co-editor of the *Medical Press.*

Doctor Kiernan was mustered in as the assistant surgeon of the Sixty-ninth New York Infantry, a three-month regiment, on April 20, 1861, but he resigned on May 22nd (*Phisterer*). His record for the next ten months is not clear but it is believed that he served with General Fremont in Missouri. He was commissioned surgeon with the rank of major of the Sixth Regiment Missouri Cavalry on March 11, 1862 to date from March 1st (*Mo. Adj. Gen.*). However, on March 7th, at the Battle of Pea Ridge, he had been wounded by a musket ball which passed through the right leg above the ankle, fracturing the tibia (*Nat. Arch.*). For seven weeks he was treated in hospitals in Cassville and St. Louis.

In May, 1863, Kiernan was again wounded. During a scout with cavalry from Port Gibson, Mississippi he was shot in the shoulder, thrown from his horse, left for dead in a swamp, and taken prisoner (*Moore*). The bullet lodged in the left lung and was not removed (*Nat. Arch.*). He escaped by night two weeks later with information of value to General Grant at Vicksburg. Surgeon Kiernan resigned again on May 24, 1863 (*Mo. Adj. Gen.*).

Here Kiernan's record once more becomes hazy. It is stated that he became a colonel of U. S. colored troops (*Phisterer*). In any event, he was appointed brigadier general of volunteers on August 1, 1863 (*Heitman*). At the end of that month he was listed as being in the Department of the Gulf (General Banks) commanding three batteries in the Nineteenth Corps (*O.R. 58*). At about the same time he reported to Adjutant General Lorenzo Thomas, who was organizing negro troops at Vicksburg (*O.R. 59*). In the Fall of 1863, he contracted malaria at Milliken's Bend, Louisiana. He came before a board of surgeons in November and was granted a sick leave of absence on account of malaria and the fresh breaking out of his wound (*Nat. Arch.*). He did not rejoin, but resigned on February 3, 1864 for disability, and his appointment as brigadier was not confirmed by the senate.

Doctor Kiernan never recovered his health. After serving briefly as a surgeon for the pension bureau, he was sent to Chin-Kiang, China as the consul. He was forced to resign in 1867 because of persistent malaria. During these years, he received a pension of $16.67 per month for a two-thirds disability from the debility of malaria and the old gunshot wound of the lung, which impaired respiration and caused occasional hemorrhage. He died in New York City on November 27, 1869 at age thirty-two, from congestion of the lungs and intermittent fever. Six months before his death an application for an increase in his pension had been disallowed on the basis that his disability was not permanent (*Nat. Arch.*). He left a wife and child.

In summary, this foreign-born, recent medical graduate, after two combat wounds, abandoned the medical service for the infantry. A test of his military capabilities was prevented by wounds and disabling disease. The reason for his early promotion to the grade of a general officer is not apparent in the record, but it was probably owing to his willingness to command Negro troops. His postwar life was soon terminated by service-incurred disease, and the depth of his interest in medicine is unknown.

19. Brevet Major General Nathan Kimball, U.S.V.

The military career of Doctor Nathan Kimball was the most varied and among the most important experienced by these thirty-three physicians. He was born at Fredericksburg, Indiana of Revolutionary forebearers on November 22, 1822 (*B.D.A.; D.A.B.; Kimball; Washburn*). His father was a merchant who shipped (like

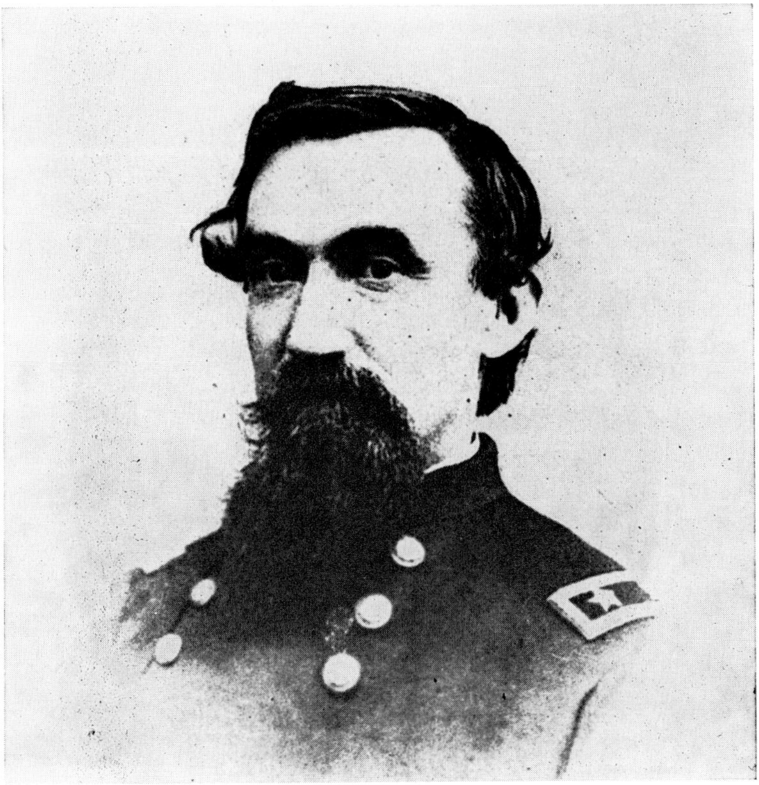

Brevet Major General Nathan Kimball, U.S.V.

Abraham Lincoln) country products to New Orleans on flatboats at a time when eastern markets were still inaccessible. He died on the Mississippi River during a trip in January, 1828 and was buried in Arkansas. The boy, Nathan, was thus orphaned at age six, his mother having died earlier, and he was raised by a grandfather, working on a farm. He attended the common schools, a country seminary, and Asbury University (now Depauw) for two years. From 1840 to 1843, he taught school and worked on farms in Iowa, and during the following year he read and practiced law. From 1844 to 1846, he studied medicine and practiced with Doctor Alexander McPheeters, and thereafter he practiced on his own. He married the sister of his preceptor in 1845. He recruited an Indiana company for the war in Mexico and, as its captain, served for one year. At Monterey, he suffered from the "bloody flux," and at Buena Vista he was thrice struck by bullets. When he applied for a pension in 1850, he still had a chronic diarrhea and, although he was not disabled, he wrote that "I am sure that I deserve a pension as much as others" (*Nat. Arch.*). After his discharge at New Orleans in June, 1847, he practiced medicine at Fredericksburg, Indiana until the Civil War (*Washburn*).

In April, 1861, Doctor Kimball recruited a company and became its captain, and on May 21st he was appointed the colonel of the Fourteenth Indiana Infantry by Governor Morton. The regiment was rushed to General McClellan in West Virginia, where it fought in several engagements that summer (*O.R. 60, 61*). In the spring of 1862, it was assigned to the division of General James Shields. At the battle of Kernstown, Shields was wounded and Colonel Kimball was left in the command. On March 23rd, he inflicted on Stonewall Jackson one of the few defeats he ever experienced (*O.R. 62*), and Kimball was made a brigadier in April (*Heitman*). The division subsequently joined McClellan's Army of the Potomac, with which it fought well at Antietam and Fredericksburg. Kimball's name became associated with two historical sites—the "sunken road" at Antietam and Marye's Hill at Fredericksburg, where the colonel in charge of the burial detail later stated that Kimball's men lay nearest the stone wall (*O.R. 63*). Kimball's superior at Antietam commended him " . . for a display of courage never surpassed"

(*O.R. 64*). The casualties in his small brigade in these two battles were respectively 639 and 520 (*O.R. 65, 66*). The latter figure includes General Kimball, who was shot through the thigh by a canister ball and in the groin by a shell fragment (*Gibbon; Nat. Arch.; O.R. 66*). The thigh wound involved much soft tissue and had not fully healed after eight months. When he was able for field duty, he was assigned to Grant at Vicksburg (*O.R. 67*). All of his subsequent service was in the two major western departments.

General Kimball, with a division, had a minor role at Vicksburg (*O.R. 68, 69*), but soon thereafter he was sent to Arkansas with a division of the Sixteenth Corps (*O.R. 70*). Eventually, he came into the Army of Arkansas of General Frederick Steele at Little Rock. In December, 1863 he went to Washington, where President Lincoln gave him instructions on encouraging the pro-Union people in Arkansas (*O.R. 71, 72, 73, 74, 75, 76*). Later Steele relieved Kimball from duty in the department in one of the nastiest episodes to be written into the *Official Records* (*O.R. 77, 78*). During this period, Kimball was involved at Fort Smith with Union General (and doctor) Blunt while Confederates Gano and Robertson, also physicians, were near by.

General Kimball got back into the main stream of the war in 1864 as a brigade and a divisional commander in Thomas' Army of the Cumberland, then advancing under Sherman toward Atlanta. Before the Fall elections, he was sent home to Indiana to help combat the disturbances of the Knights of the Golden Circle (*O.R. 79*). His men fought well in the battles of Franklin and Nashville (*O.R. 60*), and he was recommended for promotion for gallant and meritorious conduct in the battle of Franklin, for the skill, intelligence, and efficiency with which he had handled his command in the conflicts around Nashville, and for personal gallantry (*O.R. 81*). The commission of major general by brevet was given him in February, 1865. After the surrender he led troops in Texas for the war threatening in Mexico (*O.R. 82*) until he was mustered out in August, 1865.

Doctor Kimball did not return to medicine but he entered politics. He was elected the Indiana State Treasurer in 1866 and 1868 and a legislator in 1872. In 1873, he was appointed by President Grant to be Surveyor General of Utah. President Hayes appointed him postmaster at Ogden, a position he held by successive reappointments until his death in January, 1898. He had been in poor health for several years, but had done some writing on his part in the war.

As a general officer in the field in wartime, Doctor Kimball was moderately able and successful. As a brigadier, he appears better than some of the major generals. He served under a number of competent superiors in three major theatres and was liked and supported by them all but one. Only Steele, himself an undistinguished professional, was unhappy. His military correspondence is voluminous, and he is mentioned about three hundred times in the *Official Records,* nearly always creditably. The special representative of the war department at Vicksburg, Mr. Charles A. Dana, not a military man but a pretty shrewd observer although inclined to make hasty judgments, wrote to Secretary Stanton that " . . He is not so bad a commander as Lauman, but he is bad enough; brave, of course, but lacking the military instinct and the genius of generalship" (*Dana*). This subjective evaluation seems unfair when judged by the official records. Moreover, it is not in accordance with Lincoln's "cloud of witnesses." Thus, Kimball had under his command at one time or another over forty-eight different regiments from twelve states. Many of these regiments later had their histories published and most of these soldier-historians left only favorable comments.

In his voluminous war record, not a hint is found that this man was a physician. He made no comments on the health or sanitation of his commands or on the care of the wounded after battle. At one time, out of a regimental enrollment of 909, only 300 men were fit for duty because of a prostrating diarrhea (*Kepler*). After the battle of Kernstown, his senior surgeon complained of being suddenly left with 400 wounded but with inadequate supplies and organization (*O.R. 83*). However, the responsibility for this bad situation seems to fall on General Shields more than on Kimball, who had only recently taken over.

In summary, this teacher, lawyer, physician, and politician achieved his greatest success in yet another profession in two wars, the military, despite the lack of formal training. He did not return to medicine, and the record as a whole seems to show a weak interest in this field. Few other general officers had service in six major war theaters. To this wartime military record must be added his performance of two unusual political chores—in Arkansas for President Lincoln and in Indiana for Governor Morton.

20. Brevet Brigadier General Daniel Leasure, U.S.V.

Daniel Leasure was born in Madison, Pennsylvania on March 18, 1819 (*Bates; Bates*). His paternal ancestors had come to America from Switzerland, where they had gone as Huguenot refugees. He had an academic education, and graduated from the Jefferson Medical College in 1846 (*Atkinson*). He practiced first in Darlington, Pennsylvania and then in New Castle, serving also in the local militia.

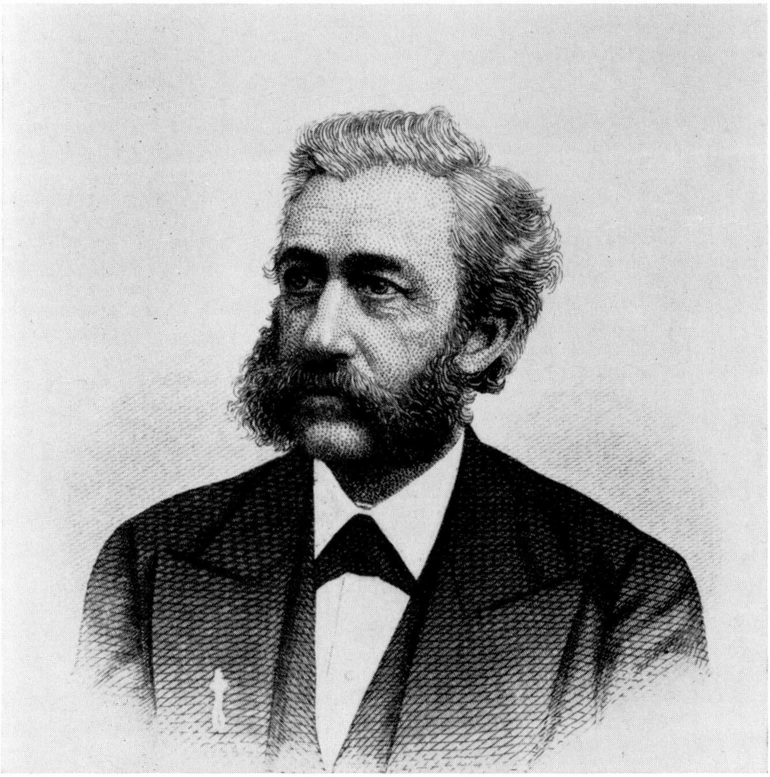

Brevet Brigadier General Daniel Leasure, U.S.V.

Doctor Leasure entered the army on April 25, 1861 as a captain in the Twelfth Pennsylvania Volunteers—a three-month regiment (*Leasure*). He served also as the regimental adjutant and as an acting assistant adjutant-general on the brigade staff of General James S. Negley. At the end of three months, he was authorized by Secretary Cameron to raise a regiment, and he was mustered in as the colonel of the One Hundredth Pennsylvania Volunteers at Pittsburg at the end of August (*Leasure*). Not having state authorization from Governor Curtin, the commissions of the officers were delayed, in some cases until after they had fought in two battles and some of them were dead. For the same reason, the regiment was not at first assigned a number so it was known as the Roundhead Regiment, and eventually it was given a high number. Raised in the southwestern counties of the state, it had many descendents of followers of Cromwell. The regiment, sent to the Department of the South, fought at Hilton Head in November, 1861 and at James Island in June, 1862. Soon thereafter they were transferred to the Ninth Corps, whose fortunes and numerous misfortunes they shared to the end. They were engaged at Second Bull Run, inactive at Antietam, transferred to Kentucky with Burnside and then to the support of Grant at Vicksburg. They were besieged at Knoxville that Fall, and were back in the Army of the Potomac for the campaigns of 1864 and 1865. During nearly all of this period, Colonel Leasure had led a brigade and on a number of occasions he had temporarily been responsible for a division (*O.R. Index*). He was mustered out at the expiration of his term of service on August 31, 1864. On April 18, 1865, he was made a brigadier general by brevet, a grade whose duties he had in actuality performed for over two years. The implication of his failure to be promoted earlier and retained in service as a brigadier is that he lacked political influence, and he had recruited a regiment in 1861 without state authorization but on the authority of Secretary Cameron, a Pennsylvanian soon discredited.

Colonel Leasure was twice wounded in battle. At Second Bull Run on August 29th his son was wounded while serving on his staff, his own horse was shot, and he was struck in the left lower leg (*Leasure; Nat. Arch.*). Securing another horse, he rode to a field hospital. Because of the many waiting wounded, he waived his turn on the dressing table and the next morning the hospital was gone. Consequently, his wound was first dressed on September 2nd in Philadelphia by Doctor Samuel Gross, who later certified that because erysipelas had set in the ball could not be removed (*Nat. Arch.*). He was out of service for about two months. The bones were not fractured. Colonel Leasure was again wounded in battle at Spotsylvania on May 12, 1864 and was sent to a hospital in Philadelphia. The nature of this wound has not been found. He had some degree of disability when he left the army in August, and he later received a pension for partial disability.

Doctor Leasure resumed practice at New Castle but he moved to Allegheny in 1870 and to St. Paul, Minnesota before 1879. Here, he died on October 4, 1886. He had been a member of the Pennsylvania Medical Society and the American Medical Association. Over a period of forty years, he published many medical papers chiefly in the *American Journal of the Medical Sciences,* the *Northwestern Lancet,* and in the *Transactions of the Minnesota Medical Society.* Most of them were reports of instructive medical, surgical, or obstetrical cases. As early as 1852, he clearly recognized a mixed epidemic of cases of puerperal infection and erysipelas, some of them transmitted by the attending physicians (*Leasure*). The writing is concise, lucid, and fluent. He also published on some interesting military experiences (*Leasure*). His official military correspondence, while not voluminous, shows the same clear style (*O.R. Index*). It suffers from gaps because post-action reporting was often omitted in the Ninth Corps. Certainly he was not seeking the attention of his superiors.

Doctor Leasure is the only physician among the thirty-three recognizable as such from the military records. This is not because the morbidity and mortality were lower in his command but because he occasionally applied his medical knowledge. Thus, after an engagement at Secessionville, South Carolina on June 16, 1862, in which the brigade casualties were heavy, Colonel Leasure voluntarily rendered valuable surgical assistance to the young regimental surgeons (*Bates*). And, after the capture of Jackson, Mississippi in July, 1863 he wrote (*O.R. 84*):

> "I trust it may not be deemed out of place in this report to speak of the fidelity with which the surgeons of their commands discharged their duties to the wounded. To their untiring efforts I have no doubts we are largely indebted for the small ratio of deaths after such very serious wounds as were most of those received at close quarters on the 11th; and, further, to express my astonishment and regret at the almost total deficiency of necessary medicines and stimulants placed at their disposal."

Whether this bold criticism came to the attention of General Sherman is not known. As usual, Sherman was travelling light.

Doctor Leasure left no known statement on why he chose the infantry. Surely it was not because of any attractive prior experience in the militia. His writings from before the war leave no doubt that he was deeply interested in medicine and had ability. His war record shows administrative ability and powers of leadership. At one time or another, at least nine different regiments served under him in brigades and many more in his divisions. Such comments as were left about him by inferiors, superiors, and regimental historians are all complimentary. But in the infantry, he accomplished nothing that could not have been done equally well by hundreds of others. Medical and organizational talent of his caliber was often deficient in the medical department. His personal experience with surgical neglect at Second Bull Run was unusual only in that the patient had high rank. The physician who traced some cases of puerperal sepsis to transmission by humans could have, one supposes, traced the cause of some of the sharp outbreaks of camp diseases to the contaminated food and water or to mosquitoes.

21. Major General Mortimer D. Leggett, U.S.V.

Mortimer Leggett was born on a farm near Ithaca, New York on April 19, 1821. He was educated at the Kirkland Seminary. When he was sixteen, his parents, members of the Society of Friends, moved as pioneers to Geauga County, Ohio, where he spent two more years on their farm (*C.A.B.; D.A.B.; Leggett; N.C.A.B.; Reid*). After studying at Western Reserve College, he was admitted to the bar in 1844, and he received the M.D. degree at Willoughby Medical College in 1844 or 1845. He became the Superintendent of

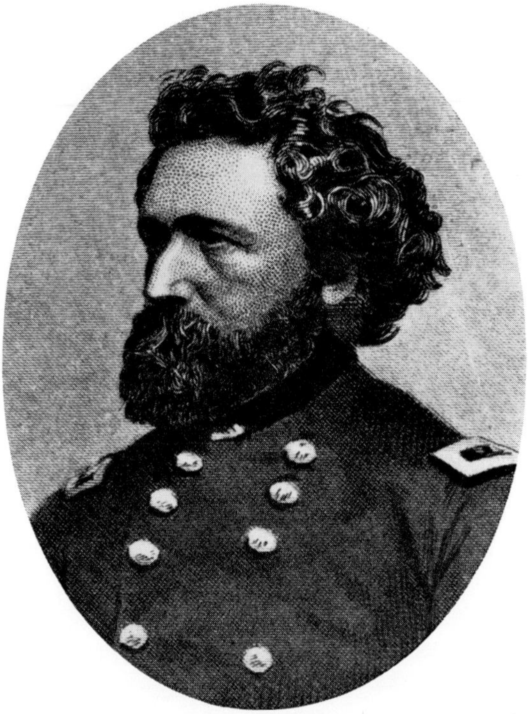

Major General Mortimer D. Leggett, U.S.V.

Schools at Akron in 1846 and at Warren, Ohio in 1849, establishing at Akron the first free graded school system west of the Alleghenys. In 1850, he opened a law office at Warren, and from 1855-1857 he was Professor of Pleading and Practice in the Ohio Law College. He moved to Zanesville in 1857, where he practiced law, superintended the public schools, published the Zanesville *Courier,* and had an interest in a machine works.

Leggett went to the West Virginia Campaign in 1861 as a volunteer aide to McClellan. On the basis, presumably, of this brief training he was authorized by Governor Dennison to recruit a regiment. In January, 1862, 940 men from the southeastern counties rendezvoused at Zanesville, with Leggett as the lieutenant colonel, to organize the Seventy-eighth Ohio Volunteers. When they arrived at Fort Donelson on February 15th, at the end of the brief siege, Leggett already commanded the regiment as colonel. From this time to the end of the war, his fortunes were joined with those of the Army of the Tennessee, successively under Generals Grant, Sherman, McPherson, and Howard. His corps commanders were usually Logan or Blair. From the middle of 1862, he led a brigade, in 1863 a division, and on several occasions he temporarily had the Seventeenth Corps. He was promoted to brigadier general on November 29, 1862, to brevet major general on September 1, 1864 (and ordered assigned to duty in that grade by the president (*O.R. 85*)), and to major general on August 21, 1865, all in the volunteer service (*Heitman*). He resigned in September, 1865. One of his notable exploits was the capture of a hill with a commanding view of the enemy's works, two and a quarter miles from Atlanta, on July 21st (*O.R. 86*). "Leggett's Hill" became a focal point in the bitter Battle of Atlanta on the following day. His divisional casualties in the North Georgia Campaign, from June 10 to September 10, 1864, were 1,420 (*O.R. 87*).

General Leggett did not escape uninjured. It is alleged that he was wounded in the hand, thigh, head, or trunk at least five times, but only one wound is adequately documented (*C.A.B.; Nat. Arch.*). These wounds were: At Shiloh, where he also had three bullet holes in his clothes (*Stevenson*); at Corinth on May 16th, where his horse was shot and he injured in the fall, but he mounted another and was soon wounded; at Bolivar on August 30, 1862, in an engagement with Generals Armstrong, Jackson, and Forrest; at Champion Hill; and at Vicksburg (*Nat. Arch.*).

At Vicksburg, in the crater at Fort Hill on June 25th, he was struck by a piece of wood splintered from a head-log by a rebel solid shot. The fragment "marked" him from the left shoulder to the right hip. He was unconscious for a while and vomited blood for several days. Pebbles and gravel were picked from the flesh of the abdomen, which was bruised and the integuments and muscles torn. When the dressings were removed, protruding bowel at the umbilicus disclosed an ugly umbilical hernia. This bothered him during the war but did not prevent his performance of duty. It persisted until his death on January 6, 1896, after a five-day illness, but whether it was the cause of his death was not recorded although death was said to have been service-incurred. At his request, this hernia was not recorded in his service record lest it interfere with his military career, but it was widely known at the time that he had been internally injured. In 1887, he was awarded a pension for disability resulting from a traumatic hernia.

General Leggett's wartime medical history is equally incomplete. He was sick a number of times and the inference from the context is that these diseases were acute and chronic diarrhea, probably dysentery. After the fall of Fort Donelson, he was made the provost-marshal by Grant at the adjoining town of Dover (*O.R. 88*). Here, great filth and stench had accumulated and some Confederate dead had been buried less than a foot deep (*Stevenson*). His regiment promptly came down with sickness, accompanied by fits of vomiting. Colonel Leggett too was prostrated, and it was feared the lieutenant colonel would die. Leggett was still severely sick and unfit for duty when the regiment disembarked at Crump's Landing on the Tennessee River on March 18th. From April 11th to May 16, 1863, General Leggett had a leave for unstated reasons (*O.R. 89*). Another similar leave was recorded for March-April, 1864. He was away sick on a surgeon's certificate of disability in August, 1864 (*O.R. 90*). At Pocotalige, South Carolina on January 15, 1865, he was sent home to save his life from a "severe chronic disease" (*O.R. 91*: *Nichols*). He returned to duty at the end of March. Leggett stated that he suffered from chronic diarrhea for several years after the war, from which he at one time lost much weight, but he eventually recovered (*Nat. Arch.*).

Leggett resumed his law practice at Zanesville. In 1871, he was appointed the Commissioner of Patents by President Grant but he resigned after four years. With two sons, he practiced patent law in Cleveland, accepting cases from as far away as the Rocky Mountains. He refused political office although he was a Republican, the party then in power. He served on the board of education, and had large manufacturing interests. He was married in 1844 and in 1879. He had four sons and a daughter, only the latter surviving him.

Despite his meager training, it is clear that General Leggett was a competent military leader, although he lacked dash and aroused little enthusiasm. Among these physician-generals he ranks with

Crawford, Kimball, Anderson and a few others of the best. Most of his superiors were able men and they all wrote well of him and recommended promotions. He had high moral standards. It is said that he did not drink, smoke, chew, swear, or play cards, and that drinking and card-playing were prohibited at his headquarters (*Reid; Wood*). His adjutant, however, testified that he had obtained liquor for the treatment of the internal injuries of his general at Vicksburg (*Nat. Arch.*). In his capacity of brigade or divisional commander, at least twenty-two different regiments came under his leadership and many of the historians later left favorable comments.

Nothing in the military record indicates that this man was a physician. In fact, in its first eleven months of service his regiment had about a dozen cases of smallpox (*Stevenson*), then the only preventable communicable disease. All men were supposed to have been vaccinated and some of these victims probably had not been. As the colonel, he could have required vaccination. He later wrote that as a physician he had fully understood the character of a traumatic umbilical hernia. This knowledge did not suffice, however, to cause him to go to the rear.

Colonel Leggett early left the Seventy-eighth Ohio for higher commands, but this regiment made a good average record, and it ended its career with Sherman and Leggett at the Victory Parade in Washington. It had travelled over 4,000 miles on foot, 3,000 by railroad, and 2,600 by water—a total of 9,600 miles. Its losses were (*Stevenson*):

Killed in battle	90
Wounded	200
Missing in action	30
Died of disease	225
Discharged for disability	295
Deserted	70
Transferred to the Invalid Corps	31

In summary, this man was successively a lawyer, physician, educator, editor, soldier, governmental bureau head, and business man. It is probable that he never practiced medicine, but he won distinction in four other professions. His investment in medicine was slight, and we do not know why he made even this commitment, or ignored it later.

22. Brevet Brigadier General Charles E. Lippincott, U.S.V.

Doctor Charles E. Lippincott reported in at Camp Butler near Springfield, Illinois, in August, 1861, with a company of men he had recruited at the invitation of Governor Yates to preserve the Union consequent to the disaster at Bull Run in July (*Elliott and Way*). He was about thirty-seven years old, and had been practicing in Chandlerville, Illinois (*Ill. Adj. Gen.*). He had graduated from the Illinois College and the St. Louis Medical College. Married in 1851, he had gone to California in 1853. There he had served in the senate, helped to keep the state free-soil, edited a paper, and killed an opponent in a duel.

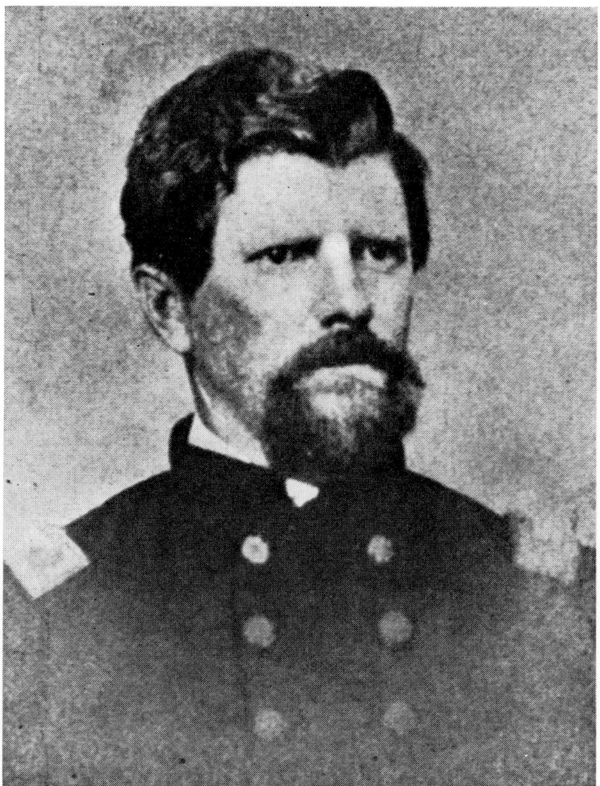

Brevet Brigadier General Charles E. Lippincott, U.S.V.

Doctor Lippincott was elected the captain of the company on September 2nd (*Heitman*), and on the 18th they started for the front in Missouri as a part of the Thirty-third Illinois Infantry Volunteers. On March 1, 1862, Captain Lippincott was elected the lieutenant colonel of the regiment, and on September 17th he became the colonel, a position he held until the end of the war, when he was made a brigadier general by brevet in the volunteers.

The Thirty-third Illinois proved to be one of the war's many hard luck regiments. It suffered few combat casualties but many from disease contracted in the swamps of Arkansas, Mississippi, Louisiana, and on the coast of Texas. It was known as the "Normal" or "Teacher" regiment because it contained many teachers, and had been recruited by President Charles E. Hovey of the Illinois State Normal University, Bloomington. One company of less than a hundred had thirteen college graduates. Hovey had witnessed First Bull Run as a civilian and had been invited by President Lincoln to help the cause. Lippincott served with the regiment in the unrewarding campaign across northern Arkansas to Helena on the Mississippi in 1862. Doctors Bussey (case 6) and Kiernan (case 18) were also in this campaign. In 1863, the Thirty-third came into the Thirteenth Corps at Vicksburg. With that ill-fated unit, they served in the Teche country of Louisiana, at Aransas Pass and Fort Esperanza in Texas in 1864, and in the District of La-Fourche in Louisiana. Finally, they had a part in the Mobile Campaign in the last weeks of the war. Except for the first two assaults at Vicksburg in May, 1863, they were in no major action, but they guarded rear areas and helped gather cotton.

Colonel Lippincott was characterized by the regimental historians as brave, generous, and alive to the welfare of the men but unable to perform even simple maneuvers with the regiment. He was a rare conversationalist and story-teller, and excelled in writing good English. His military correspondence is too scanty to justify a fair opinion on his abilities (*O.R. Index*). In appearance, he was five feet and eight inches tall with a light complexion and black eyes (*Nat. Arch.*).

As in the case of many other physicians, the health record of Colonel Lippincott is incomplete because he often treated himself. A surgeon certified that Lippincott had several attacks of fever in November, 1862 and earlier (*Nat. Arch.*). About May 1, 1863, in the rear of Vicksburg, he had attacks of chills and fever and of diarrhea. Despite treatment by the regimental and brigade surgeons, he gradually became worse so that in July he had to be sent back from the second Jackson expedition to a hospital because of weakness (*O.R. 92*), and he was soon invalided home. By July 1st, he had hemorrhoids, attributed to the diarrhea, and a fissure in ano was recorded some years later. He had relapses of malaria in 1864, and chronic diarrhea resulting in general debility that led to long sick leaves that year (*Nat. Arch.*).

In the assault of May 22nd on Vicksburg, Colonel Lippincott was struck on the foot by a minie ball (*O.R. 93*). He was knocked from his horse, the heel was blasted from his boot, his heel and half the sole were bruised, and his leg was paralyzed for a time. He was taken to the hospital and treated for shock. There was no residue from this injury.

Doctor Lippincott returned to his home at Chandlerville near Springfield a semi-invalid. He tried to resume the practice of medicine but found himself unable to do a day's work because of weakness. He had constant diarrhea and any exertion brought on fever. In 1885, he was awarded a pension for full disability resulting from "Malarial poison, chronic diarrhea and piles." He had delayed so long in applying for the pension because he had other means. He was defeated for congress but was the doorkeeper of the House of Representatives for a while and the auditor of Illinois for two terms. Eventually, he became the superintendent of the Soldier's Home at Quincy. Here he died of "general paralysis" on September 11, 1887. He was buried at Springfield. That diagnosis did not then carry the specific etiological connotation it has since acquired. His paralysis was certified as being the result of his chronic diarrhea and piles. Mrs. Lippincott survived until 1896, and as "Mother Lippincott" was the popular and adored matron of the hospital at the Soldier's Home (*Elliott and Way*).

It seems clear that Doctor Lippincott was a popular colonel but militarily not particularly able or ambitious. Poor health may have interfered with his vigor and development. Quinine was available for his malaria but there was nothing effective for either bacillary or amebic dysentery. His experiences on the frontier in California suggest that his interest in medicine was weak and that a spirit of adventure took him into the infantry. This regiment had no physical examinations on induction.

23. Brevet Brigadier General Benjamin Chambers Ludlow, U.S.V.

Benjamin C. Ludlow was born near Cincinnati, Ohio in 1831 (*B.D.A.; Reid*). He studied at Carey's Academy and Kenyon College, and graduated in medicine after two years of study at the University of Pennsylvania in 1854 (*Ludlow; U. Pa.*), writing his thesis on "The Formation of Callus." After practicing in New York City for one year, ill health compelled him to seek a milder climate, so he spent a year in California and three in Mexico. In

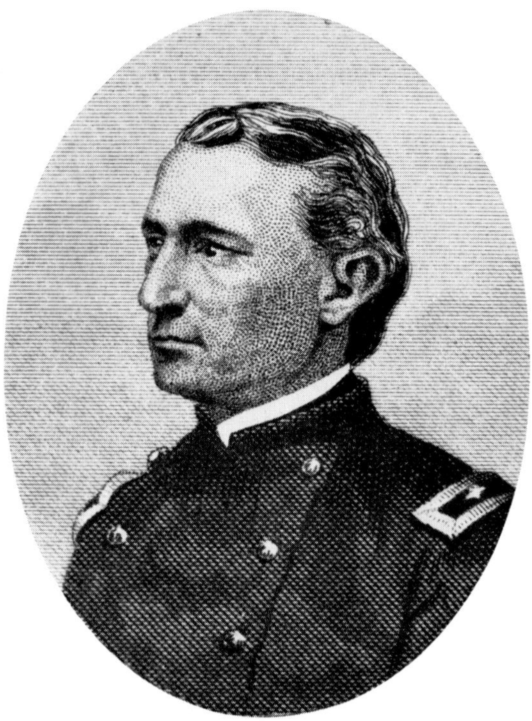

Brevet Brigadier General Benjamin C. Ludlow, U.S.V.

1859, he was appointed an assistant surgeon at the Longview Lunatic Asylum in Cincinnati.

In 1861, Doctor Ludlow recruited a company of cavalry, only to be told that additional cavalry would not be required as the four regiments already accepted would be enough. He then became a lieutenant and a captain in Fremont's Hussars at St. Louis, participating in the campaign in southwestern Missouri that fall and winter and in Arkansas in early 1862. There is an unverified statement that he was wounded (*B.D.A.*). The Hussars were consolidated with the Fourth Regiment Missouri Cavalry when Fremont lost the departmental command, Ludlow becoming a major (*Mo. Adj. Gen.*).

Major Ludlow had various staff positions with Generals Dix (*O.R. 94*) and Meade in 1863 (*O.R. 95*) and, possibly, with Hooker (*B.D.A.*). In 1864, he was on the staff of General Ben Butler of the Army of the James, as an inspector of cavalry (*O.R. 96, 97*). In August, he was placed in charge of cutting the canal at Dutch Gap (*O.R. 98*), a sizeable engineering project for which he had no obvious qualifications. On recommending him for promotion, General Butler wrote "Maj. B. C. Ludlow, of the additional staff, for gallant and meritorious conduct in maintaining for many days his position under fire at Dutch Gap and for meritorious conduct in leading his troops in the charge on Spring Hill, August 30, 1964. This last gentleman is entitled to great praise for silent and quiet endurance and the example he has set for the men, having done more than any other officer to inspire the colored troops with steady coolness under fire. He has had his quarters at Dutch Gap twice shot to pieces, almost under him, by the enemy's shell." On October 28, 1864, he was promoted to brigadier general by brevet (*Heitman*), and in December he was assigned to duty in this grade by the order of the President (*O.R. 99*). In 1865, he had various small rear area cavalry and district commands (*O.R. 100, 101*). No record is found that he was in a major campaign or battle. He was a brother-in-law of Secretary Chase but he did not use this connection for military preferment.

Doctor Ludlow resigned in August, 1865. He resumed the practice of medicine, but poor health led to frequent changes in location (*Nat. Arch.*). His war medical record shows an attack of boils in 1863, a severe bronchitis, and hemorrhoids; the latter two diseases caused some disability after the war. He lived in Cincinnati until 1869, in Champaign County, Illinois until 1870, in Texas until 1885, in Paxton, Illinois "for the prairie air" until 1887, and in Berkeley, Kern City, and Los Angeles, California until his death on January 10, 1898. He suffered at times from frequent colds, a morning cough, and throat troubles. Climatotherapy, including the mountain air on several occasions, were palliative at best. His lung disease, finally diagnosed as chronic bronchiectasis, was recorded as the cause of death together with pneumonia. He left a wife and five children.

In summary, this physician with a prewar record of impaired health served throughout the war creditably in various staff and cavalry capacities. After the war he resumed the practice of medicine when his health permitted, but continuing lung disease led to a number of changes in location. His eventual death appears to have been caused by a service-augmented if not incurred disease.

24. Brevet Major General William Linn McMillen, U.S.V.

William McMillen was born at Hillsboro, Ohio, on October 18, 1829 (*B.D.A.; McMillen*). In 1853, after two years of study, he graduated from the Starling Medical College in Columbus, where he practiced until the war came. Like other young physicians, he offered his services for the Crimean War to the Czar of Russia through the Russian Minister in Washington, and was accepted in May, 1855. He had duty with an army of 100,000 men at Helsingfors, Finland, and in a hospital of 1,700 beds at Tavastehus. After traveling to St. Petersburg and in Western countries, he resumed practice in Columbus in 1856. In 1860-61, he edited the *Review of Medicine and Surgery* at Columbus.

Doctor McMillen became the surgeon of the First Ohio Infantry on April 17, 1861 (*Heitman*). They were sent to the field immediately and, before their three-month term had expired in August, they had fought at Bull Run. McMillen then became the surgeon-general of Ohio, serving until Governor Dennison was succeeded by Governor Tod (*Reid*). He was authorized to recruit an infantry

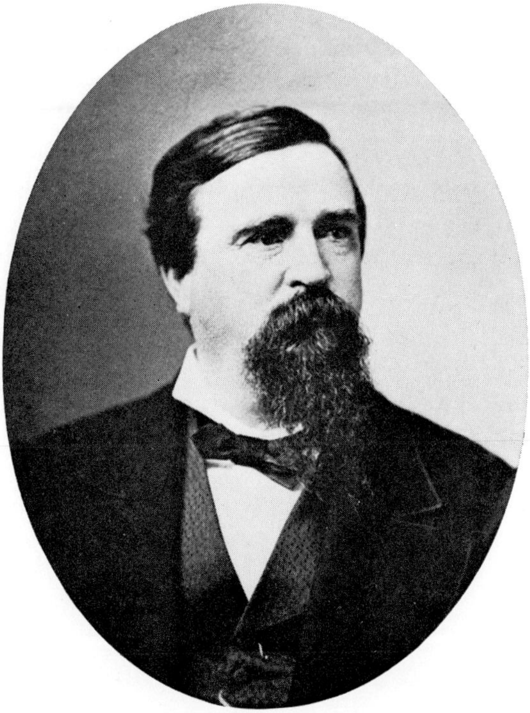

Brevet Major General William L. McMillen, U.S.V.

regiment, which was mustered in on August 14, 1862 as the Ninety-fifth Ohio Volunteers with Doctor McMillen as its colonel. Without training or even complete organization, they were routed in the battle of Richmond (Kentucky) two weeks later (*O.R. 102*). In this battle, Colonel McMillen was shot in the hand by a rifle ball and was taken back to Columbus for treatment. For this wound, he received a pension for one-half disability after the war (*Nat. Arch.*).

When the regiment was again ready to take the field, it was sent to the Army of the Tennessee for the Vicksburg Campaign of Grant. They were never heavily engaged but they were the first regiment to enter Jackson (*O.R. 103*). Afterward McMillen was in command of a brigade at various times. In 1864, he was in three of the expeditions sent from Memphis against Forrest, including the disastrous affair of General Sturgis', in which he led the infantry division of three brigades (*O.R. 104*). In June, 1864, he came into the command of General Andrew J. Smith, under whom his fortune improved. Under Smith, he went on the Tupelo expedition against Forrest (*O.R. 105*), into Missouri against Sterling Price, and against Hood at Nashville in December. In this, his first and only major battle, he performed admirably so that General Thomas wired the President (*O.R. 106*): "Brevet Major General Smith . . carried the salient point of the enemy's line with McMillen's brigade, of McArthur's division, capturing sixteen pieces of artillery, two brigadier-generals, and about 2,000 prisoners." General McArthur in turn telegraphed the President a day later (*O.R. 106*): "I respectfully ask, as an act of justice and honor fairly won, that Col. W. L. McMillen, . . be appointed brigadier-general;" Smith and Thomas endorsed with approval and the promotion was made by brevet. At the end of the war, he was awarded the higher rank of brevet major general. General McMillen was active under General Canby at the fall of Mobile, had various district commands during the early part of the occupation, and was mustered out in August, 1865. By chance, he had been in several hard campaigns but in few battles. No evidence is found in his military record that he was a physician.

Doctor McMillen did not return to medicine but he became a cotton planter in Louisiana and later a politician. He was a delegate to the state constitutional convention in 1868, a state senator from 1870-72, and a United States senator in 1872 and in 1873 but he was not allowed to take his seat. He was the postmaster at New Orleans under President Hayes and the surveyor of the port under President Harrison. He died in Columbus, Ohio on February 8, 1902.

In summary, after serving for three months as the surgeon of one regiment, Doctor McMillen became the colonel of another. His leadership in the infantry was creditable but not distinguished except at the battle of Nashville. For this service, he was eventually promoted to major general by brevet. He did not return to practice but became a planter and politician in the deep south. Whether a partly disabled hand consequent to a war wound played any part in this decision is not known.

25. Brevet Brigadier General Abram O. Miller, U.S.V.

Abram Miller was born in Madison County, Ohio on October 3, 1827 (*Magee*). His parents moved to Indiana in 1830 where both died in 1833, and the boy was taken into the home of a farmer. He graduated in medicine at the University of Louisville in 1856, at a time when Doctors Samuel Gross, Yandell, Flint and others comprised a famous faculty. He was practicing in Lebanon, Indiana when the war began (*Nat. Arch.*). His first wife died in 1853, a second one in 1857, and he was remarried in 1862, four children surviving from this union. He had no interest in politics but regarded himself as a Jacksonian Democrat and a strong Unionist although he had voted for Buchanan and Douglas.

After the attack on Fort Sumter, Doctor Miller quickly raised a three-month company and, as its captain, joined the Tenth Indiana Volunteer Infantry on April 25, 1861 (*Heitman; Shaw*). The

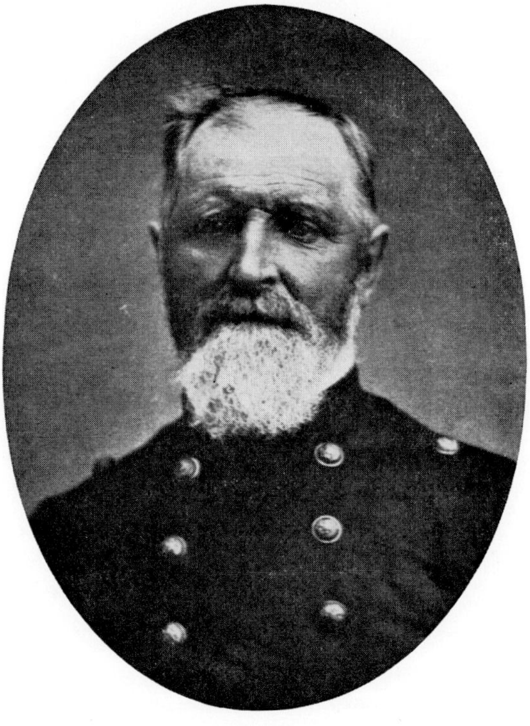

Brevet Brigadier General Abram O. Miller, U.S.V.

regiment had service in West Virginia under McClellan before its term of enlistment expired in August. Miller had made a reputation as a brave, calm, discreet officer. He reenlisted in September and became the major. To help win the battle of Mill Springs in January, 1862—the first major Union victory—his men fired sixty to seventy-five rounds apiece (*O.R. 107*). He led the regiment as its lieutenant colonel from April, 1862 under Buell in Kentucky and Tennessee. In August, Governor Morton appointed him the colonel of the new Seventy-second Indiana, and he joined this regiment at Lebanon, Kentucky on August 23rd. They had assignments in Kentucky and Tennessee but missed the battles of Perryville and Stone's River. At Chickamauga they had an important role (*O.R. 108*). Late in 1863, Colonel Miller was given the command of a new brigade of mounted infantry, equipped with Spencer repeating rifles, in the Department of the Cumberland. Operating as cavalry, the brigade contended with Wheeler's horsemen on several occasions. In 1864, they were in Sherman's cavalry in North Georgia, and they were among the army components left behind by Sherman in November to help General George Thomas in Tennessee. At Louisville in the winter of 1864-65, they were re-equipped, but too late to fight at Nashville. However, they came into General James H. Wilson's cavalry corps for the spring campaign of 1865 into Alabama. At Selma, on April 2nd, in battle with Forrest, Colonel Miller was shot in the thigh (*O.R. 109*). He was carried along in a carriage to Montgomery. Because of threatening gangrene, he was left here when Wilson moved on into Georgia, and he came into the hands of Confederate surgeons as a prisoner (*Nat. Arch.*). However, he was released when Montgomery was soon reoccupied by Union forces, and when his old regiment passed through Nashville on their way home in June, they found him there, still unable to walk or ride a horse, but glad to help muster them out of service (*Magee*). He never recovered completely from this wound. The ball had entered anteriorly at the junction of the middle and lower thirds of the thigh, passed obliquely downward, and made its exit posteriorly just above the popliteal space.

Colonel Miller had experienced heavy service and fought in many engagements, but by chance early in the war and because he commanded mounted infantry and cavalry later, he had not been in a major battle prior to the one at Selma in 1865. Already in 1864, he had long led a brigade, and he had been recommended for promotion to the corresponding rank on several occasions. The recommendation was renewed by General Wilson, and the promotion to brigadier was finally made in brevet grade to date from March 13, 1865. He was mustered out in June. His health had been good apart from an attack of camp diarrhea lasting for some months in 1863, disabling at times, and the leg wound.

Doctor Miller returned to Lebanon and intermittently practiced medicine for some years (*Nat. Arch.*). His health deteriorated steadily, and he was at times incapacitated by pain in his wound, loss of sight and hearing, and other ailments. On several occasions, he had young men reading medicine in his office. He also served as clerk of the court and cashier of a bank. By 1870, he was nearly deaf and blind on one side. He died on April 25, 1901. The cause of death was given as pneumonia complicating a gunshot wound of the thigh and a concussion injury of the head from an exploding rebel shell.

In view of Colonel Miller's education and experience as a physician, the medical record of his Seventy-second Indiana regiment is of some interest (*Magee*). He took command at the end of August, 1862 at Lebanon, Kentucky. By October 7th all were lousy. By October 20th, diarrhea raged, and a virulent measles had broken out. They were eating rotten maggoty meat and their hard tack contained white worms. Scurvy appeared in November. Severe colds were now so common that the picket line could be located at night by the coughing. In late November, more than half the regiment was sick. As it moved from place to place on various guard assignments, it left a trail of sick and dead; the dead in the first six months totalled ninety-four men. They died as follows: At Jeffersonville, Indiana, 2; New Albany, 7; Louisville, 13; Frankfort, 2; Bardstown, 2; Bowling Green, 7; Scottsville, 6; Gallatin, 27; Nashville, 4; Murfreesboro, 24. In addition, 190 officers and men had been discharged. During the second six-month period, 146 more were lost to the regiment, thirty-eight of them by death. At this time, another 300 men and nine officers were sick in hospitals.

The official strength at Indianapolis had been 978 officers and men. Combat casualties had been few.

In his diary, the regimental surgeon wrote on April 29, 1863, when the regiment was encamped with Rosecrans' Army of the Cumberland at Murfreesboro, Tennessee (*Magee*):

> "This army of 40,000 is encamped on a space so small that it is utterly impossible to keep the camps clean. Thousands of dead horses, mules and offal of every description, literally cover the face of the earth inside our picket lines; and each emits a thousand stinks, and each stink different from its fellow. The weather for months had been almost one continual flood of rain, and now, as the sun comes up more nearly straight over us, and pours down its boiling rays on this vast, sweltering mass of putridity, the stinks are magnified, multiplied and etherealized until the man in the moon must hold his nose as he passes over this vast sea of filth."

Certainly, nothing in this health or sanitation record suggests that the colonel was a physician.

General Wilson, Miller's last superior and one of the bright lights to shine from the war, thought highly of him. Wilson wrote that the colonel was steady, quiet, intrepid, unassuming, unobtrusive, big, solid, and sound. He was serious and thoughful, and looked like a country doctor on his rounds (*J. H. Wilson*). A biographer concluded (*Kemper*): "He was a good man, a good physician, and a patriot. He deserves a shaft as high as Bunker Hill monument."

In summary, this physician without military training promptly entered the army as a captain of infantry and quickly rose to the command of two regiments and eventually a brigade. He went by way of the mounted infantry to the cavalry, in which he won his stars as a brigadier by brevet. He suffered a prolonged camp diarrhea, and a gunshot wound in the last weeks of the war left some permanent disability. On returning to the practice of medicine, he was handicapped by a progressive invalidism which he attributed to a war-incurred cerebral concussion by a rebel shell. Since he was regarded as a good physician and regimental commander, the bad health record of his regiment must reflect the ignorance of the times.

26. Brevet Brigadier General Albert James Myer, U.S.A.

Albert J. Myer was born at Newburgh, New York on September 20, 1827 (*B.D.A.; J. W. Brown*). His parents soon moved to western New York. His mother died and he was raised by an aunt. In 1847, he graduated at Hobart College and entered the medical department of the University of Buffalo. Here, he finally graduated in 1851, supplementing the aid of his aunt by employment as a telegraph operator (*Nat. Arch.*). This skill led to the subject of his thesis, which was on "A New Sign Language for Deaf Mutes" (*Myer*), and to his lifelong interest in the problems of communication. For impaired health, he now spent several months on a farm in Canada, that winter in South Carolina, and some time in Florida, where he recovered. It is said that he practiced medicine during this period.

In 1854, Doctor Myer was appointed an assistant surgeon in the army and ordered to the southwestern frontier. From observing

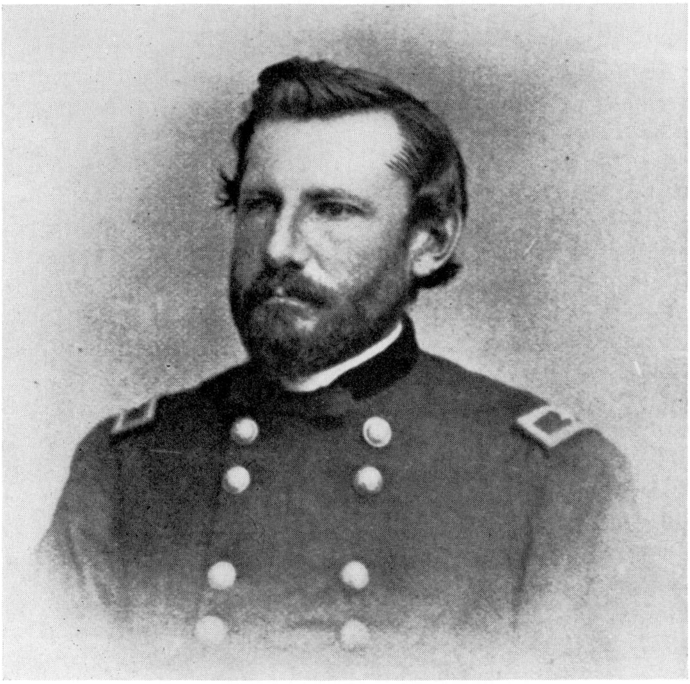

Brevet Brigadier General Albert J. Myer, U.S.A.

the Indians, he became interested in rapid communication by signals. Assigned to special signal duty from 1858-60, and aided by a special congressional appropriation of $2,000 for equipment, he devised a signalling system for flags by day and torches by night. The war department in 1860 created a signal department with Myer as signal officer with the rank of major (*Heitman*). The system was tested in New Mexico in 1860-61 against the Navajos.

In the war, Major Myer organized and commanded a signal camp at Fort Monroe, served as aide to General McDowell at First Bull Run, established signal courses and camps of instruction, and acted as the signal officer with the Army of the Potomac under McClellan. In 1863, the Signal Corps was organized by an act of congress, and Myer was appointed the chief signal officer with the rank of colonel by the president (*Nat. Arch.*). Secretary Stanton failed to send this appointment to the senate for confirmation and it lapsed in 1864, whereupon Major Myer was replaced and assigned to routine duties in the field. In the Department of the Gulf, he arranged the terms of surrender of Fort Gaines in 1865. For a time, he was without assignment. However, in 1866, with the support of Grant he was restored to the position of chief signal officer, and in 1868 he was belatedly made a brevet brigadier general, U.S.A. for distinguished services, to date from March 13, 1865. He was promoted to the full grade in 1880.

In the meantime, Myer's interests broadened and expanded, ever farther from medicine. He wrote a manual of signals that went through several editions (*Myer*). In 1870, he was assigned the duty of making meteorological observations available to the public through an extensive telegraph system, and eventually this influence was felt in every seaport and hamlet in the land. Under his supervision, 5,000 miles of electric telegraph lines were built (*Nat. Arch.*). He helped establish an international system of simultaneous meteorological observations. He represented the United States at international meteorological congresses in Vienna in 1873 and Rome in 1879. In the midst of his greatest usefulness he died, still in the service, at age fifty-two of Bright's disease at Buffalo on August 24, 1880. He left a wife and six children. He had been awarded an LL.D. degree by Hobart in 1872, and a Ph.D. by Union College in 1875.

It is not known whether his renal disease dated from the illness of 1851.

In summary, it is evident that the major interest of this physician was early turned from medicine to the problems of mechanical communication techniques. His potential contribution in the war was impaired by friction in the war department, but he must be credited with founding the signal corps and, later, aiding in the development of the weather bureau. It is probable that his lifelong intense interest was aroused by his experience as a telegrapher while a medical student and by his medical thesis on manual communication by deaf mutes.

27. Brigadier General Lucius Bellinger Northrop, C.S.A.

Doctor Northrop, a personal friend of Jefferson Davis, became the highly controversial Commissary-general of Subsistence of the Confederate Army. He was born in Charleston, South Carolina on September 8, 1811, and graduated at West Point in 1831, twenty-second in a class of thirty-three (*Cullum*). Most of the next eight years were spent as a lieutenant of infantry or dragoons on the western frontier at Fort Gibson in the Indian Territory. In 1835-37, he had an extended sick leave for a bullet wound of the knee accidentally inflicted by himself (*Hay*). In 1839, he was wounded during the Seminole War in Florida, and he never returned to active duty (*B.D.A.; D.A.B.; Warner*). He studied at the Jefferson Medical College in Philadelphia but did not graduate. In 1848, he was dropped from the army for practicing medicine in Charleston, but he was soon not only reappointed but also promoted through the influence of Senator Jefferson Davis. He remained in private practice in Charleston while on furlough until the war. He resigned from the army in January, 1861 soon after his state had seceded.

In 1861, Doctor Northrop was appointed the commissary general by Davis, and he served until February, 1865, when he was relieved under the pressure of an act of the Confederate congress. The rank of brigadier general was awarded him in November, 1864 but the appointment was not submitted to the senate for approval. Among the charges brought against him were inefficiency, inadequate feeding of prisoners, and grasping for power. He, in turn, blamed his

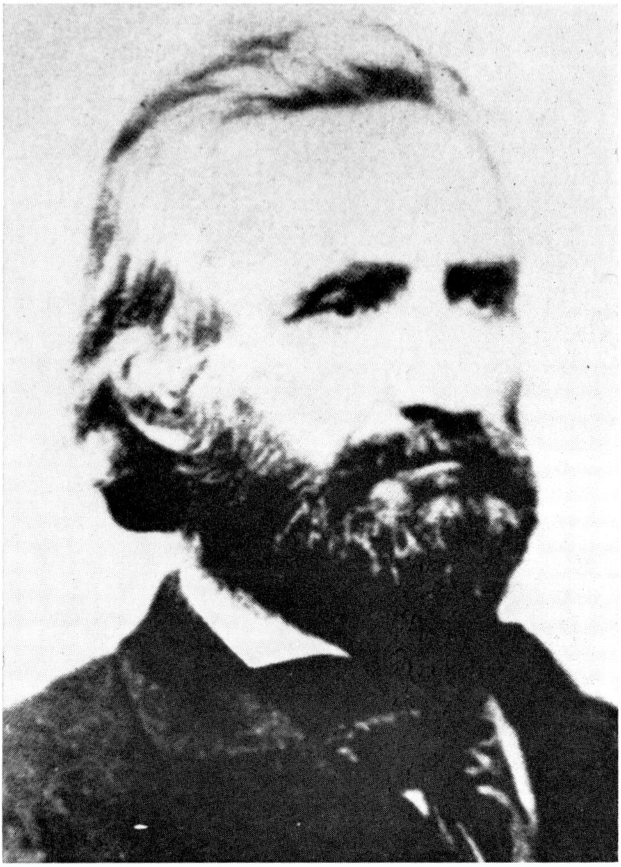

Brigadier General Lucius B. Northrop, C.S.A.

troubles on insufficient funds, an inadequate transportation system, and the unpopularity resulting from the need for impressment and price-fixing to obtain food (*Hay*). He was the most unpopular officer with the army and the congress next to Bragg, but he lasted so long through the support of Davis. Some unfortunate personality traits seem to have contributed to his troubles. Some defenders held him blameless (*Evans*). In connection with his official position, his military correspondence in the *Official Records* is enormous (*O.R. Index*).

After the war, Northrop was arrested by the Federal authorities for having starved prisoners, but no formal charges were brought and he was paroled after some months (*Nat. Arch.*). He retired to a farm near Charlottesville, Virginia and, in self-defense, did some writing, both public and private. After a stroke of paralysis in 1890, he entered a soldier's home at Pikeville, Maryland, where he died on February 9, 1894.

In summary, this West Point graduate studied medicine after having been wounded and disabled in Indian warfare, and he practiced for about twenty years. In the war, he became the unpopular and controversial Confederate commissary general. He did not resume the practice of medicine.

28. Brigadier General Jerome Bonaparte Robertson, C.S.A.

Jerome Robertson was born in Woodford County, Kentucky, on March 4, 1815 (*D.A.B.; Evans; Warner*). He was orphaned at an early age and apprenticed to a hatter in Kentucky and St. Louis from age twelve to seventeen. During this time, he had only three months of schooling. At age seventeen, he became a pupil and assistant of Doctor M. W. Harris, first in St. Louis and later in Owensboro, Kentucky. In 1835, he graduated in medicine at Transylvania University and entered practice. A year later he raised a company of volunteers for the Texas independnce movement, but they arrived there after the war was over. However, he practiced medicine in Washington County and Independence, Texas for over thirty years, the beloved physician of a large area. He took a part in Indian campaigns, held office as coroner and in both houses of the Texas legislature, and was a delegate to the secession convention in 1861.

Doctor Robertson entered the military service by election as a captain on August 3, 1861 (*Nat. Arch.*), and soon went to Virginia with the Fifth Texas Infantry. In June, 1862, he was the colonel of the regiment and by November he was a brigadier general in the command of Hood's Brigade of Texans. He fought in most of the heavy battles of 1862 and 1863 in the East, and he went with Longstreet's Corps to fight at Chickamauga and Knoxville. In the winter of 1863-64, he was arrested by Longstreet and brought before a court martial on charges of conduct prejudicial to good order and

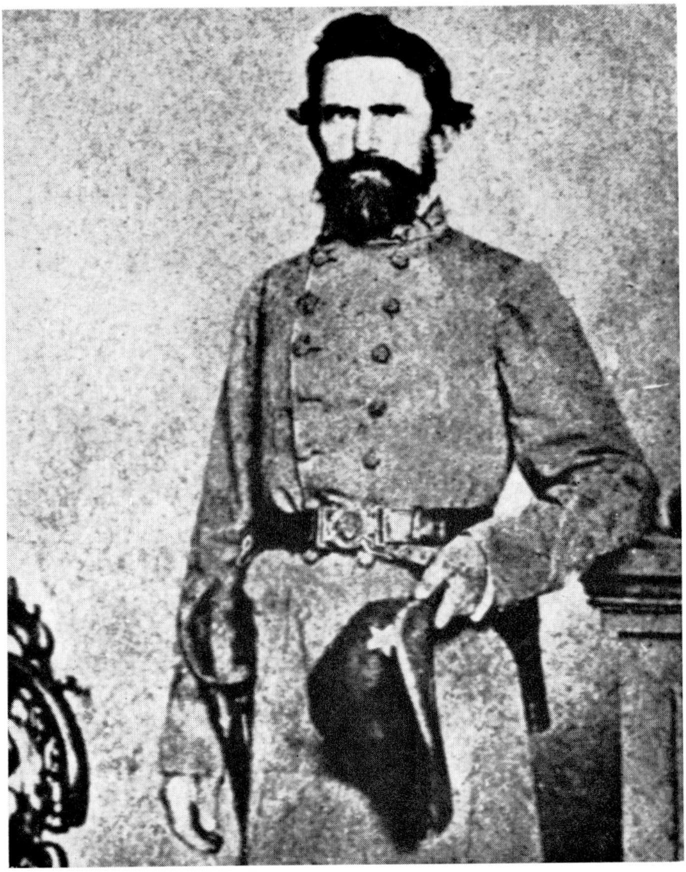

Brigadier General Jerome B. Robertson, C.S.A.

military discipline (*Nat. Arch.; O.R. 110*). He had criticised the high command too freely, was found guilty, and was reprimanded. Among other things he had tried, through political influence, to have the Texas Brigade, depleted to 677 men after two years and a half, sent home for rest and recruitment (*O.R. 111*). In June, 1864, he was sent to Texas to command the reserve force of the state (*O.R. 112, 113*). There he ended the war in charge of a brigade (*O.R. 114*).

Robertson was wounded three times. At the battle of Gaines' Mill in June, 1862, still a colonel, he was slightly wounded in the shoulder (*Nat. Arch.; O.R. 115*). Two months later, at Second

Bull Run, he was again wounded (*O.R. 116*). At Gettysburg, while he was leading the Texas Brigade in the Devil's Den, he was struck above the knee (*O.R. 117*). The disabilities from these wounds were temporary. However, the woundings show that he directly shared the hazards of battle with his men.

Nothing in his military record suggests that Robertson was a physician. His men were not especially well cared for. An inspection report on his brigade of five regiments on November 14, 1862 records 440 men barefooted, about two-thirds of the men badly clothed and shod, and over 200 rifles missing or in bad order. Perhaps a brigadier should not be held responsible for the supply and ordnance situation in his command at that period of the war. He was the father of Brigadier General Felix H. Robertson, the last surviving Confederate general officer and the only Confederate general credited to Texas actually born in that young state (*Warner*).

Doctor Robertson returned to his practice in Texas. Later, he held appointive political positions and was interested in railroad development. He died in Waco on January 7, 1891.

In summary, this physician entered the infantry directly from civilian life as a junior officer and became a general officer in about sixteen months. After a period of heavy service he was relegated to a secondary position. He was wounded in battle three times. He returned to medicine after the war. A son also became a general officer.

29. Brevet Major General Robert Kingston Scott, U.S.V.

Robert Scott was born in Berks County, Pennsylvania on July 8, 1826 (*B.D.A.; C.A.B.; D.A.B.; N.C.A.B.; Nat. Arch.; Warner*). His grandfather served in the Revolution, his father fought in 1812, and he would fight in two wars. In 1842, he went to Starke County, Ohio, and attended a Central College for a while. He spent nineteen months with a Pennyslvania regiment in the Mexican War, reaching the grade of captain (*Heitman*). Thereafter, he studied medicine in Navarre, Ohio and at Starling Medical College, Columbus, in 1850. He then mined gold in California, where he also practiced. After prospecting in Mexico and in South America, he settled in Florida, Ohio in 1851, soon married, and practiced medi-

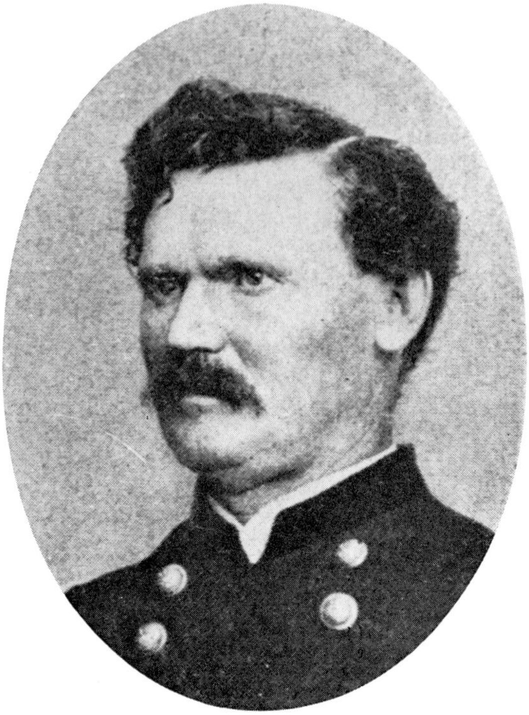

Brevet Major General Robert K. Scott, U.S.V.

cine until 1857. It is said that his suppression of a cholera epidemic gave him much local prestige (*D.A.B.*). Profitable investments in real estate enabled him gradually to withdraw from medicine and engage in merchandising. When he entered the military service, he was a physician and merchant at Napoleon, Ohio (*Nat. Arch.*).

Doctor Scott became the lieutenant colonel of the Sixty-eighth Ohio Volunteer Infantry on November 30, 1861, and its colonel in the following July. This regiment at Fort Donelson joined the forces that eventually became the Army of the Tennessee, and its entire service was with that army. It was assigned, finally, to the Seventeenth Corps, which it accompanied through Georgia to the sea and up to Raleigh. Colonel Scott led a brigade during most of the time after 1862. It is noteworthy that throughout most of his career he followed one step immediately behind and under General Mortimer Leggett, another Ohio physician-general described elsewhere in this study. Scott was promoted to brigadier general of volunteers on January 12, 1865 and to brevet major general on December 2, 1865. Like many others, he had some hard campaigning but he participated in few major battles. He left little military correspondence (*O.R. Index*), making only one post-action report (*O.R. 118*). Perhaps this should be blamed on General Leggett and others for careless administration. All of the few comments made about him in the Official Records are complimentary.

General Scott has no record of wounds or sickness but he was injured. He was captured at Atlanta on July 22, 1864 before the battle began (*O.R. 119*), and exchanged in about nine weeks. While being taken to prison in Charleston, South Carolina, he attempted to escape by jumping at night from a moving train near Macon, Georgia (*Nat. Arch.*). He fell down an embankment, injuring his back, breast, right leg and knee. When he later applied for a military pension, he stated that he had suffered from spinal disease, trouble in his back and knee, and heart disease ever since. However, on recommending Scott for promotion in December, 1864 at Savannah, Brigadier Leggett had stated that his health was excellent.

General Scott remained in the army until July, 1868. For nearly three years, he was an assistant commissioner of the Freedman's Bureau in South Carolina. He won wide support and, after resigning, he was elected the Republican governor of the state in 1868 and re-elected by a sizeable majority in 1870. During his second term, however, he was charged with various abuses. These included the fraudulent overissue of state bonds, bribing the legislature with public funds, and manipulating printing contracts and the stocks of the Blue Ridge Railroad (*D.A.B.*). He defeated impeachment charges for misconduct. After leaving the statehouse, he settled in Columbia as a real estate agent. In 1876, he supported the state Democratic ticket, declaring Negro suffrage a mistake. When the Democrats came into power in 1877, he left the state (one biographer said "prudently" (*D.A.B.*)), and returned to Napoleon, Ohio, where he engaged in real estate operations. A quiet life was interrupted in 1880 when he was brought to trial for shooting and killing a young drug clerk whom he believed responsible for making his young son drunk. He was acquitted of manslaughter. Scott was stricken with apoplexy in May, 1899 and he died at Napoleon on August 13, 1900. The cause of death was given as "Paralysis" (*Nat. Arch.*).

The record is conflicting in a number of respects on this physician, whose life was so adventurous if not turbulent. He was six feet and one inch tall, brown haired, grey eyed, and had a florid complexion. One critical biographer of his carpetbagger days wrote that he was " . . subject alike to alcoholic and female allurements" (*D.A.B.*). In contrast, General Leggett, himself a man of high morality, wrote into the record that he was a man of correct habits, great energy, and indomitable will, who was capable and gallant (*O.R. 120*). Nothing in his military record suggests that this man had a medical education, and he left no known statement on the reason for his choice of service.

30. Brevet Brigadier General William P. Wainwright, U.S.V.

William P. Wainwright was born in New York City on June 10, 1818. He attended the University of the City of New York, graduating in medicine (*A.P. Smith*). Not wishing to practice, he went to Europe for military studies in Berlin. When the war came, he was a member of the militia of Dutchess County and "a person of leisure" (*Nat. Arch.*).

Wainwright became the major of the Twenty-ninth New York Infantry on June 17, 1861 at their solicitation (*Smith*). This was a regiment of Germans organized by Adolph Von Steinwehr (later brigadier general), and Wainwright was known to speak that language. In December, he took a sick leave for "bilious catarrhal fever" (*Nat. Arch.*). After the Battle of Cross Keys in the Shenandoah Valley in June, 1862, Wainwright was commissioned the colonel of the Seventy-sixth New York. He found the regiment undrilled, but within two months they fought at Second Bull Run (*O.R. 121*). The regiment was there reported to have been thoroughly disciplined and to have held its position with determined obstinacy. Two weeks later, Colonel Wainwright was wounded in the arm at South Mountain, and he was cited for gallantry and good conduct (*O.R. 122*). His horse was killed. He rose, tied a handkerchief around his arm, gave the order to fire, and emptied the six barrels of his revolver

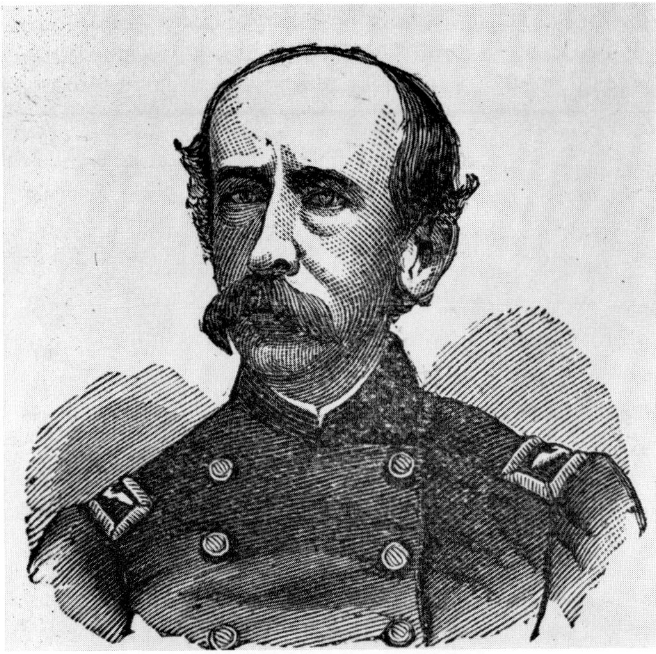

Brevet Brigadier General William P. Wainwright, U.S.V.

at the enemy, who fled (*Smith*). The colonel then addressed the regiment, after which he went on sick leave. When he rejoined in November, his arm was not yet healed. The regiment was present but took little part in the battles of Fredericksburg and Chancellorsville. En route to Pennsylvania, Colonel Wainwright was sick, and he received the surgeon's permission to fall to the rear because of malaria. Five days later (on June 17, 1863), he left on a sick leave. On June 19th, he was appointed the provost-marshal of the District of Columbia, but he resigned on the 25th, and took no further part in the war (*O.R. 123*), although the resignation was not accepted until 1864 (*Phisterer*). He was made a brigadier general by brevet after the war, to date from March 13, 1865.

General Wainwright was an invalid for the rest of his life. He lived chiefly at Rheinbeck but died in New York City at age seventy-seven on October 17, 1895 of acute bronchitis and asthenia (*Nat. Arch.*). The nature of this incapacitating, long-standing illness is uncertain. A catarrhal bronchitis had begun in April or May, 1863.

It was accompanied by a persistent cough, great physical reduction, and hoarseness with inability to speak above a whisper. Since this is not the picture of malaria alone, it is probable that he had also a major chest disease, possibly tuberculosis.

This seems to be yet another case of service-incurred disability. General Wainwright's military correspondence is scanty, but all comments and actions in the *Official Records* are creditable (*O.R. Index*). The Seventy-sixth thought him an able and earnest officer. He drilled hard, was strict, but attended carefully to the needs of the men, and they were sorry to see him leave (*Smith*). On the first Sunday in camp, the chaplain being absent, the colonel invited a captain, who was also a minister, to conduct the services. When he refused, the colonel himself conducted them. As far as is known he never practiced his first profession, that of medicine. Regardless of whether this was because of ample personal means or some other reason, it seems to indicate a low interest in this profession.

31. Brevet Brigadier General Mark Fernald Wentworth, U.S.V.

Mark F. Wentworth was born into an old colonial family on March 14, 1820 at Kittery, Maine. Here, he would live for most of his life and practice medicine for over forty years (*Houston; Stone; Wentworth; Whitman and True*). He attended the local public schools for four months each winter to the age of twelve while working on his father's farm. After his father died in 1832, he attended high school and an academy half time. He began the study of medicine at age twenty-one with Doctor Trafton of South Berwick. From 1842 to 1844, he attended medical lectures at Dartmouth College. He then became the chief clerk at the Portsmouth navy yard from 1845-1849, and a clerk with the state valuation commission at Augusta thereafter. He then studied medicine at the University of Pennsylvania and, after practicing briefly at South Boston, he moved to Kittery. In 1854, he helped to organize a company of militia—the Kittery Artillery—which he commanded. In politics, he was an ardent Republican, and as a delegate to the Chicago convention in 1860 he supported Lincoln.

When the war began, Doctor Wentworth was appointed chief

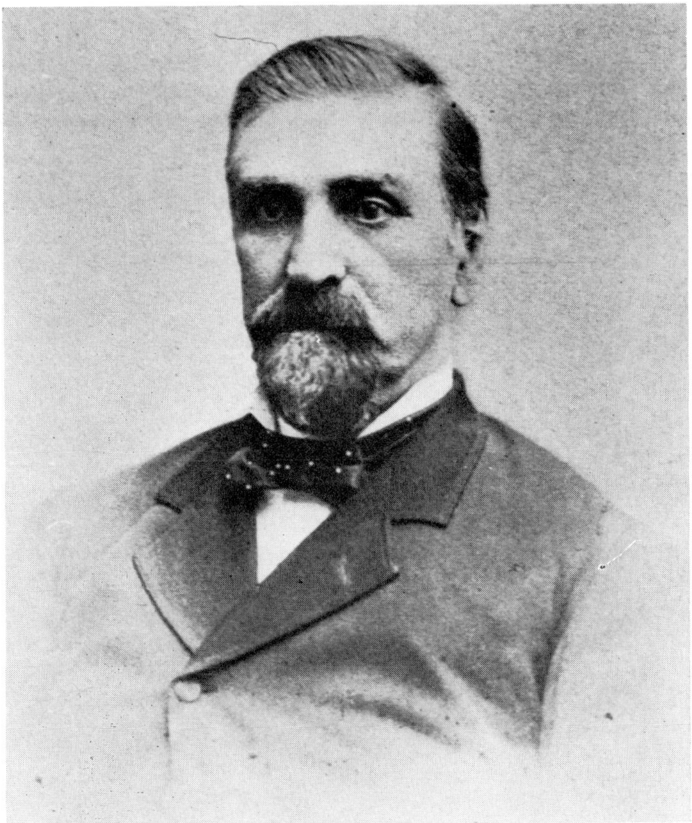

Brevet Brigadier General Mark F. Wentworth, U.S.V.

of staff to Governor Hamlin with the state rank of lieutenant colonel. His Kittery Artillery garrisoned Fort McClary in the emergency from April until June, 1861. He organized the Twenty-seventh Maine Infantry Volunteers in 1862 and was elected the lieutenant colonel in September and the colonel in the following January (*Heitman*). The regiment served its term of enlistment of nine months in the defenses of Washington, south of the Potomac, without being in battle. Wentworth was later awarded a medal of honor for volunteering to remain on duty after the term of enlistment had expired until the outcome of the battle of Gettysburg was known. In 1864, Colonel Wentworth organized the Thirty-second Maine and, as its colonel, took them to the front. They joined the Ninth corps of the Army of the Potomac in May after the Richmond campaign had begun. This time Colonel Wentworth was in the field less than three months. He became ill at Fredericksburg on May 23rd and was sick until the 26th at least (*Houston*). He went to the hospital sick again on June 19th. The diagnosis for these illnesses has not been found. In the attack through the mine crater on July 30th, he was shot through the side and carried from the field. The ball passed through the "body" but further details have not been found. He was taken north, but recovery was slow and he was discharged for disability on October 18, 1864. Later he was awarded the grade of brigadier general by brevet to date from March 13, 1865.

For the rest of his life, Doctor Wentworth held a series of state and federal elective and appointive positions and sinecures in addition to practicing medicine occasionally. He retained an interest in politics and was a delegate to the Republican national convention in 1868, but he failed of election to congress in 1873. He was reappointed the storekeeper at the navy yard, had two terms in the state legislature, and was a member of the board of inspectors of state prisons for four years. Under appointment by President Harrison, he was the surveyor of customs at Portland from 1891-95. He died at home at Kittery on July 12, 1897, leaving a wife and two daughters.

Doctor Wentworth held the confidence of the people of his community well enough so that he was able to recruit and command regiments in 1862 and 1864. His abilities as a military leader were, however, never fully tested because of the nature and short periods of his two field services. The second was ended by a wound received in his first battle, but he was congratulated by General Bartlett for being the only colonel to lead his men into the Crater (*Chase*). The Official Records contain no military correspondence of his, and he is mentioned only in the tables of organization (*O.R. Index*). There is nothing in his military record to suggest that he had a medical education.

It is of historical interest that the Twenty-seventh Maine, composed of 949 men commanded by a physician, in its nine months of service during which it was never in battle or in really unhealthy swampy country, nevertheless lost twenty men by death, fifty-four by discharge, and eight officers by resignation. The discharges were probably chiefly for disability, some of them for conditions existing prior to enlistment and not screened out by examination.

From the pre- and post-war records it seems that Doctor Wentworth had high qualities as a citizen but that his interest in medicine was relatively weak.

32. Brigadier General Edward A. Wild, U.S.V.

Edward A. Wild was born in Brookline, Massachusetts on November 25, 1825 (*C.A.B.*). He graduated from Harvard College in 1844 and from Jefferson Medical College in 1846 (*Wild*). He served

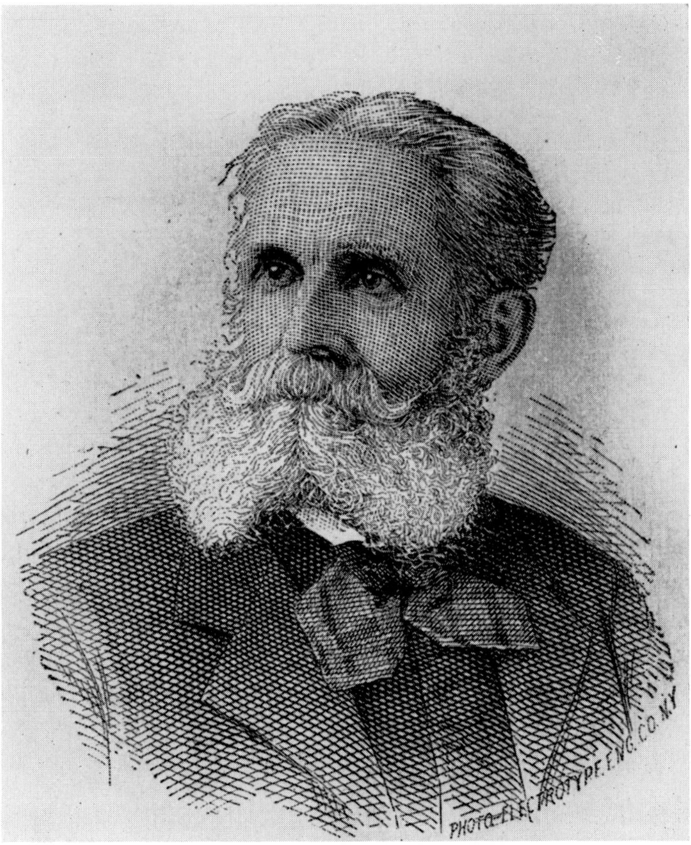

Brevet Brigadier General Edward A. Wild, U.S.V.

as a surgeon in the Crimean War (*Bowen; Schouler*), and in 1861 he was practicing in Brookline. He had been a member of the state medical society from that town since 1850.

Doctor Wild became a captain in the First Massachusetts Infantry on April 21, 1861. As a New Year's present, twenty of his Harvard classmates sent him an elegant sword (*Cudworth*). On June 25, 1862, at the beginning of the Seven Days' battles, he was shot by a bullet through the palm of the right hand; the first and second fingers were permanently disabled (*Cudworth; Nat. Arch.*).

In July, 1862, promoted to major (*Heitman*), he helped to recruit the Thirty-second Massachusetts Regiment (*Parker*). On August 21st, he became the colonel of the new Thirty-fifth Massachusetts, and he took them to the front, his arm still in a sling (*Mass. Thirty-fifth*). Three months later, in the engagement at South Mountain, his left arm was struck by a round shot just as his brother, an aide, lost an eye and General Jesse Reno nearby received a mortal wound (*Gordon; O.R. 124*). His arm was amputated near the shoulder that night (*Wild*). Healing was delayed by the repeated formation of abscesses in the stump (*Nat. Arch.*).

Despite a crippled hand and the loss of an arm, Colonel Wild was promoted to brigadier general on April 24, 1863 and sent to North Carolina to recruit a brigade of Negro troops (*O.R. 125*). In recommending him to the war department for this assignment, Governor Andrew cited as his qualifications the facts that he was the right age, a Harvard graduate, and a physician (*Schouler*). Eventually he recruited Wild's African Brigade (*O.R. 126, 127*), about 2,000 strong, but there were strong Confederate protests at his methods (*O.R. 128, 129*). In 1864, the brigade came into General Ben Butler's Army of the James. Here General Wild's career was not smooth. In June, 1864, he was arrested and convicted by court martial of insubordination, but the verdict was set aside by Butler and the judge-advocate-general (*C.A.B.; Livermore*). Again, in February, 1865, charges were filed against him (*O.R. 130*) at a time when he was in charge of a division of the Twenty-fifth Corps. General William F. Smith had judged him "entirely unfitted" to lead a colored division (*O.R. 131*). He was relieved of his field command in March, 1865 and was assigned to the Freedman's

Bureau in May (*O.R. 132*). The Confederates retaliated against Wild for having hung North Carolina troopers as guerillas (*O.R. 133*), but General Butler defended him. He was mustered out of service in January, 1866. He had seen some hard service but had not been in a major battle since South Mountain.

Doctor Wild did not return to medicine, giving as his reason his physical disabilities, for which he was pensioned. He became interested in mining, and lived for extended periods between 1876 and 1891 at a mine in Canada. He was troubled intermittently by a diarrhea thought to have been contracted in the war (*Nat. Arch.*). The record on this disease is not clear because he had always treated himself. In 1891, he went to South America with a friend to investigate mining interests. Here he had an acute exacerbation of diarrhea, from which he died on August 28th. The verdict of one writer that in his career " . . adventure was more prominent than medicine" (*Wild*) seems to be justified.

In summary, this physician who had surgical experience in the Crimean War early entered the Civil War as an infantry officer, and eventually became a brigadier general. He was incapacitated for field service by the loss in battle of one arm and the partial disablement of his remaining hand, so he was assigned to the recruiting and training of colored troops. He did not return to medicine, giving in explanation his physical disability—a reason not entirely convincing. He died of an acute enteritis superimposed on a chronic war enteritis.

33. Brevet Brigadier General Samuel Morton Zulich, U.S.V.

Samuel Morton Zulich was born at Easton, Pennsylvania, on March 1, 1842 (*Bates*). His father was an imigrant from Frankfort-on-the-Main and his mother a resident of Philadelphia. He had a classical education at Easton, and graduated at Jefferson Medical College in 1844. He was married in 1846 and a son, Philip, later served in the Forty-fifth Pennsylvania Volunteers. Zulich gave his occupation in 1861 as that of a railroad official (*Nat. Arch.*), and it is not known when he abandoned medicine.

Zulich enlisted as a private in the Twenty-ninth Pennsylvania

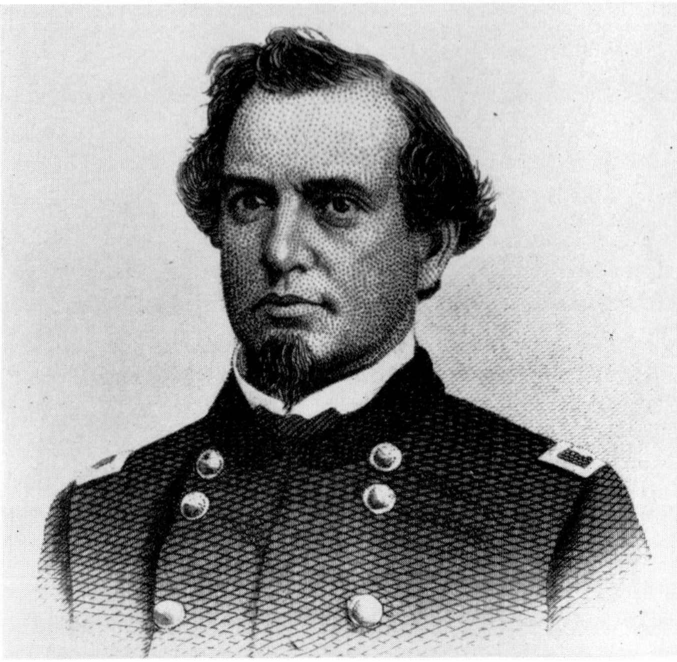

Brevet Brigadier General Samuel M. Zulich, U.S.V.

Volunteers for three months on May 15, 1861. On its reorganization as a three-year regiment, he became a captain. This turned out to be a hard luck regiment. It campaigned in the Shenandoah Valley in 1862 against Stonewall Jackson. At Winchester, it broke and many men were captured. Captain Zulich avoided capture and, as the senior officer present, he made the regimental post-combat report (*O.R. 134*). Thereafter the regiment was assigned to the Twelfth Corps, Army of the Potomac. It did not fight at Second Bull Run, Antietam, or Fredericksburg, and it was only lightly engaged at Chancellorsville and Gettysburg. With the corps under Hooker, the regiment was sent to the support of Chattanooga in the fall of 1863. Its fortunes were thereafter linked with those of Sherman. With him it went to Atlanta, to the sea, and, finally, up through the Carolinas to Washington in 1865.

Captain Zulich was promoted slowly but steadily (*Heitman*): To major in March, 1863, to lieutenant colonel in May, 1863, and to colonel in March, 1865. He was later awarded a promotion by brevet to brigadier general to date from March 13, 1865 for bravery and efficiency as an officer. He was honorably mustered out at Camp Cadwallader on July 17, 1865.

The promotions of Zulich were slow because of his occasional illness, because of the failure of the colonel to be promoted or resign, and because the regiment was not prominent in battles although it had some hard campaigning. The brigade and divisional commanders for several years were the relatively colorless Generals John W. Geary and A. S. Williams. Nevertheless, Zulich won a number of special citations. Thus, at the Battle of Lookout Mountain he arose from a sick bed " . . and by his courage and energy added fresh spirit to all. . . Ever at the front, his courage was worthy the emulation of all" (*O.R. 135*). Lieutenant Colonel Zulich was the sixth and last commander of the regiment during the four-month campaign to Atlanta in the summer of 1864, he himself having been sick earlier in the summer (*O.R. 136*). He missed the Carolina campaign in early 1865 because of illness, but he rejoined at Goldsboro on April 10th, and took part in the march to Raleigh and in the Victory Parade (*O.R. 137*). His military record and correspondence show competence at the field grade level and untested abilities above that.

Zulich contracted diarrhea near Chattanooga about November 24, 1863, and this condition persisted until his death at home in Philadelphia at age fifty-two on June 10, 1876 (*Nat. Arch.*). Upon his discharge, he was a semi-invalid but this fact is not shown in the records of the adjutant general. He worked as a real estate operator when able. During the war, he was treated only in camp except for several leaves of absence on medical certificates of disability. When he was examined for a military pension in September, 1875 he was five feet seven and one-quarter inches tall but he weighed only 119 pounds. He had formerly weighed 190 pounds. He was still losing flesh because of chronic diarrhea and diabetes, and was living on a milk diet. Death was attributed to "Pleuro Pneumonia with cheesy deposit." His physicians, Doctors James McClintock and H. James Goodman, performed an autopsy which disclosed also a cystic condition of the pancreas and large kidneys. The cystic pancreas was believed to explain the diabetes and the "fatty discharge from the bowels." The cheesy deposits were not located or described. Doctor Goodman expressed an intention to report this interesting case, but such a publication has not been found. In the absence of additional information, an etiological diagnosis is uncertain but an intervention by one of the infectious granulomas must be considered. Tuberculosis was not a rare complication of chronic and exhausting dysentery, especially after the war.

Promotion from private to general officer, change in profession from physician to general, continuation in active field service with a walking dysentery or some other disease, muster out as a semi-invalid with nothing in the military record so to indicate, and eventual death from a service-incurred condition—all illustrated by Zulich's case—were not uncommon in that war as is shown by even this small group of case reports. Thousands of men must have been unable to march in the Victory Parade up Pennsylvania Avenue because there were no relief stations along the route. The cheerful acceptance by these physician-generals of their diseases and of their often ineffective management, and their continuation in field service to the end despite partial disability reflect the spirit of the times—evidence of an acquiescence that today is sometimes hard to understand.

Chapter IV

PRE-WAR LIFE

In this chapter, the search is begun for factors in the early life of these officers that might explain their wartime choice of duty. It soon became apparent that the group of physician-generals was different from the controls in several respects.

Date and Place of Birth

The thirty-three physician-generals were born between 1802 (Brandon) and 1837 (Kiernan). Their background was, therefore, post-Revolutionary for the oldest members of the group; for many it was pioneer and immediately post-pioneer. The range in birth dates was approximately the same for the four groups.

The thirty-three future physician-generals were born in thirteen different states. Two were foreign-born: Kiernan was a native of Ireland and Elliott of Scotland. The place of birth of one (Lippincott) has not been found. The states were represented roughly in proportion to the sizes of their populations, considering the small size of the sample. The populous states of New York, Pennsylvania, and Ohio each was the birth place of five, Indiana of three, Kentucky, Maine and South Carolina each of two, and the rest were scattered. In 1837, when the youngest of these doctors was born, there were only twenty-six states. Some of these states were new and had only a small native-born population. It is clear that the origin of the physicians who became generals was not regional.

In the three control groups, the birthplace of some members was not found, but the distribution by states in the remainder was as widely scattered as in the physician-general group. New York and Pennsylvania, as the most populous, led. One or more foreign-born officers were found in every control group.

Rural *versus* Urban Boyhood

The boyhood environment was rural for sixteen of the members of Group I, urban for seven, and unknown for ten. The urban category includes several towns of sizes that today would be regarded as rural. In fact, there were no very large cities in the country at the time when these doctors were boys. Since over ninety per cent of the total population was then regarded as rural, the background was urban in an undue proportion of these physician-generals.

The same statement can be made for the members of the control general and control physician groups. The boyhood environment of too many of the matching enlistees is unknown to warrant deductions on this group. Inasmuch as the available findings were similar in the first three groups, the phenomenon of the physician-generals is not explained by the type of general environment they experienced during their formative years.

Father's Occupation

These physician-generals came from homes of many kinds. The fathers of fifteen were farmers, three were clergymen, two were physicians, and one each was a teacher, merchant, engineer, and politician. The occupation of seventeen was unknown. In Groups II, III, and IV, the occupation of even more of the fathers is unknown. However, among those on record, farmers and planters were the most common. For one or more member of each group, the father was a physician. Only a few fathers had shown an active military interest. The occupation of the fathers of the future officers does not explain the phenomenon under study.

Premedical Education

The general and premedical education of these physician-generals as a group was far above the general level, as would be expected. At least seventeen of them had attended a college or university and nine were known to have graduated. Three others were described as having had a classical, academic, or seminary education. Four more had attended public schools. One was chiefly self-educated but, his father having been a clergyman, he probably received a good education in the home. The early education of eight is unknown.

In the control groups II, III, and IV, the education is known for twenty-four, thirteen, and ten, respectively; six, six, and three had graduated from or attended a university or college. Graduates of the U. S. Military Academy numbered one in Group I, six in Group II, and three in Group III. As will be emphasized later, the number of lawyers was greater in Groups II and III than among the physicians of Groups I and IV.

Medical and Postdoctoral Education

Most of these physician-generals had the medical education of the times. This usually consisted of attendance at two series (often identical) of lectures of variable length but commonly about five months each. Twenty-five had thus attended American medical colleges and one in Glasgow (Elliott), and many of them had graduated. At least four of the twenty-five had, in addition, studied medicine with a physician before completing the lectures. The medical education of four (Anderson, Bussey, Champion, Kimball) consisted solely of study with a practitioner as far as is known. For three (Brandon, Capehart, Wainwright) the type of medical education is unknown.

Jefferson Medical College, which had the largest classes at that time, had been attended by at least four of the twenty-six, Starling and Louisville each by three, and Dartmouth, Pennsylvania, and St. Louis each by two. The remainder had attended at Harvard, Yale, New York, Cleveland, Indiana, Willoughby, Buffalo, Transylvania, Cincinnati, South Carolina, and Glasgow.

At least four (Cameron, Elliott, Wentworth, Wild) had some postdoctoral medical education, one of them going to Paris (Wild).

For the control surgeons of Group IV, medical education, known for twenty-one of them, was essentially like that of the physicians of Group I. Most of the same schools were represented and a few new ones were added. Jefferson Medical College led again with five graduates. The University of Maryland and the University of Pennsylvania each had two and the others were scattered. The Vermont Medical College, the Colleges of Physicians and Surgeons at Keokuk and in New York, the Medical College of Georgia, and Edinburgh University were among the schools additionally represented in Group IV. Four men had also some postdoctoral medical education before the war, two of them in Europe. At least five students preceded or supplemented their medical lectures by study with a physician.

From this comparison of Groups I and IV, it is apparent that the medical education was similar. Moreover, the war-time decision of the members of Group I cannot be attributed to the influence of any special school or to medical educations that were substandard for that period of history.

Prewar Medical Practice

In April, 1861 twenty-four doctors of Group I were practicing medicine part or full time. Nine were out of medicine; two (Leggett, Wainwright) had never practiced and seven had abandoned medicine and were now lawyers (Champion, Elwell), merchants (Bussey, Hillis), planter (Anderson), and railroad official (Zulich), and one (Myer) was developing the army signal service. Of the two who had never practiced, Leggett was a lawyer and Wainwright a man of leisure.

The twenty-four in medical practice were widely scattered in twelve states and the army (Crawford). Indiana and Ohio were each home to four, New York, Massachusetts, Illinois, South Carolina, and Texas each had two, while Kansas, Maine, Mississippi, Pennsylvania, and Virginia each contributed one. Most of these physicians were practicing in small towns, but five were in cities. New York City was the home of two (Elliott, Kiernan), and Charleston, Columbus, and Cincinnati each of one. Because of the method of their selection, the members of Group IV cannot be used for a comparison on these points.

Only one of these doctors was a specialist. Elliott was regarded as an ophthalmologist or oculist—which, is not clear. A greater number of specialists was found among the control physicians.

It is concluded that the geographical and the rural:urban distributions were approximately representative of the total population, but it is clear that the medical interest of many members of the group was weak.

Additional Professions or Occupations

An outstanding finding in these physician-generals is the large proportion that had one or more occupations or professions in addition to medicine. This is true even if the temporary occupations of their youth and premedical days, such as farming and teaching, are disregarded. Ten had only the profession of medicine, but the other twenty-three had from one to five additional occupations even before the war. Nine had one other occupation, ten had two more, and three had three, four, and five additional occupations respectively. In all, the twenty-three physicians had forty-one occupations in addition to medicine. To these the military profession was added during the war. Counting medicine and the military, the thirty-three physician-generals each had an average of nearly three and a half professions or occupations. After the war some took up additional professions.

The commonest second prewar occupation was that of politics. Ten of these doctors had been in local, state, or national politics. The commonest political position by far was in the state legislatures, in which capacity eight had served. Six were editors and/or publishers of newspapers (Cameron, Leggett, Lippincott), of medical periodicals (Kiernan, McMillen), or of legal journals (Elwell). Five were lawyers (Anderson, Champion, Elwell, Kimball, Leggett). Five taught or superintended schools (Elwell, Harris, Kiernan, Kimball, Leggett). Business had attracted five (Bussey, Hillis, Leggett, Scott, Zulich). Four (Myer, Northrop, Robertson, Wainwright) were military men beyond the stage of the militia or Mexican War enlisted man. Anderson, Brandon and Harris were farmers or planters. Champion had been a printer, Myer a telegrapher, Scott a prospector, and Elwell the author of law books. It is evident that many of the thirty-three had other interests and were not deeply challenged by medicine.

The physicians of Group IV, in contrast, were far more attentive to medicine. As far as is known, twenty-seven were practicing in 1861 and two more probably were also. Three had one additional interest: one (Udell) served in the Iowa senate, one (Rex) taught in a state normal school, and one (McGugin) edited the *Iowa Medical Journal* on the side; he had been in the Ohio legislature at one time. One (Martin) had been a clergyman for twenty-two years and ran a girl's school. Thus, the thirty-three together had a total of only five additional occupations. It is obvious that they were much more firmly committed to medicine. If the members of this group are taken as representative of the medical profession, then the physician-general group was distinctly atypical by this criterion.

Prewar Political Interest and Activity

The record is incomplete but it is known that at least ten of these physician-generals had held political office at the national, state or local levels. Anderson had been the appointive governor of Washington Territory. Sitting in state legislatures had been Anderson and Brandon (Mississippi), Bussey (Iowa), Cameron (Indiana), Elwell (Ohio), Dustin and Lippincott (California), and Gano (Texas). Furthermore, Blunt had been a delegate to the Wyandotte constitutional convention in Kansas, Robertson a member of the secession convention in Texas, and Anderson a delegate to the Florida secession convention and to the convention of Southern states that formed the Confederacy at Montgomery in 1861. The political affiliation, if any, of many of the Northerners is not known, but the others were divided between the Republican and the Douglas wing of the Democratic parties. Harris had been a Whig and Lippincott a Free-soiler. As far as is known, all were unionists and some were abolitionists as well. After the war, others also participated actively in politics, usually as Republicans, the party long in power. The political convictions of these doctors no doubt were a factor in their decision to enlist, but it is not known that these beliefs played a role in their decision to fight rather than to heal.

The control physicians, in contrast, had shown far less interest in politics. Only Doctors McGugin (Ohio) and Udell (Iowa) had been in state legislatures. Palmer had been a delegate to the Florida secession convention.

The political interest of the control generals, however, was nearly equal to that of the physician-generals. Generals Branch and Logan had been members of congress and Brevard, McNeil and Miller of state legislatures. Lippitt had been a member of the California state constitutional convention, and Miller a county judge, while Hartranft and Roddey were sheriffs. Four had been Democrats—Bate and Branch of the Southern wing and Hartranft and Logan of the Northern, Logan campaigning in 1860 as a presidential elector for Douglas. King and Leake were Republicans, Leake having been a delegate at the Wigwam in Chicago. After the war, several more were Republicans, that party controlling the political rewards. The record is incomplete on twenty-two, but if the six army (Brooks, Chambers, Crook, Gardner, Michler) and navy (Page) officers are omitted as being nonpolitical, the inactive or unknown group is reduced to sixteen.

The documentation is poorer on the matching enlistees. General Wagner had served in both houses of the Indiana legislature. Colonel Ward had been a member of the Confederate provisional congress, and Granbury a county judge. If the three professional military men (Clary, Gorgas, Sykes) are eliminated, a group of twenty-seven remains about whom no information is available on this point. Among the five physicians within this group, there is no record of political activity. The group includes a number of lawyers, in whom it would be strange for that period to find all political interest lacking if the record were known.

In summary, many physician-generals had a prewar interest in politics. In this respect the group was more like the controls generals than like the control physicians. Many of the physician-generals were distinctly men of action and leadership by the criterion of political activity, and for physicians they were unusual in this regard.

Migration and Travel

Many of these physician-generals had moved, or been taken as boys, westward from their place of birth, participating in the great movement of the time. Twelve of these doctors, born in eastern states and two from Europe, had moved westward. In so doing, they tended to maintain their latitude. Only two (Gano, Robertson), who had migrated from Kentucky to Texas, violated this rule. In addition, many of the nineteen who enlisted from the state of their birth had travelled west for reasons not connected with their schooling but had eventually returned home. Thus, at least four (Dustin, Lippincott, Ludlow, Scott) had been in California where they had prospected, practiced medicine, served in the legislature, published a newspaper, or thrown down other temporary roots. It is evident than some of these doctors had been restless.

The information on prewar migration by the members of the three control groups is less complete than on the physician-generals. However, it is known that at least ten of the control generals had moved westward from their place of birth, one had moved southward, and two were immigrants. McNeil had come from Nova Scotia and Sewell had been brought from Ireland. Among the control enlistees, at least seven had moved westward and one was an immigrant from Ireland (McDermont). In Group IV, seven members had moved westward, one north, and one had gone south. Doctor Milhau had been born in France.

It is uncertain that significant statistical differences exist between the four groups in this regard. Some men of all groups were typical Americans of the time in their tendency to be taken or to migrate westward. The new states beyond the Mississippi (Minnesota, Iowa, Missouri, Arkansas, Texas, Louisiana, California, Oregon) had few native-born citizens of military age (except in New Orleans and St. Louis), and even slightly older states, such as Michigan and Wisconsin, had many immigrants from the east. For example, the Second Regiment Iowa Infantry enrolled 1,669 members in its first two years of service *(Iowa Adj. Gen.)*. Only ninety-eight (5.8 per cent) had been born in Iowa. The remainder had immigrated from at least twenty-three other states and thirteen foreign countries. Ohio had given birth to 451 of them, Pennsylvania to 205, Indiana to 196, New York to 183, and so on. One hundred and seventy-six had been born abroad, with Germany, England, and Ireland contributing the most—forty-two, thirty-eight, and thirty-eight, respectively.

In contrast to migration, prewar travel had been commoner among the physician-generals than the control physicians. The latter had not gone to California, the Crimea, and elsewhere. This criterion indicates a certain restlessness and lack of firm commitment on the part of some of the physician-generals.

Prewar Military Education and Training

These thirty-three physician-generals had little or no military background. Sixteen had no prewar military training whatever, as far as is known, and the others had only a little. Doctor Blunt had been a member of the military committee of the Kansas constitutional convention in 1859. Wild and McMillen had experience as surgeons in the Crimean War; in the Civil War one began as a surgeon and the other went directly into the infantry. Crawford and Myer had been assistant surgeons in the army for some years. Doctors Bussey and Hillis began as aides to Governor Kirkwood of Iowa, serving for a few months in 1861, Leggett aided McClellan in this capacity in West Virginia, and Wentworth was the chief of staff to Governor Hamlin of Maine. Four had been in the army during the Mexican War—Anderson as a lieutenant colonel, Hillis as a private, and Kimball and Scott in grades up to captain. Robertson volunteered in the war for the independence of Texas but too late to serve; later he had fought Indians on the frontier during emergencies. The state militias had provided a little training to five—Anderson, Brandon, Leasure, Wainwright, and Wentworth. Brandon had been a major general in the Mississippi militia, but he was now fifty-seven years old, and his war record would be good but not distinguished. Wainwright had received some military training in Germany as well as in the New York militia, but his wartime record was shortened by wounds and disease. Of the thirty-three, only Northrop had been really militarily educated. He had graduated at West Point in 1831, but after eight years of experience on the frontier he had retired for disability. Neither the Military Academy nor medical lectures at Jefferson in 1840 fitted him for the important and difficult position of Confederate commissary-general. It must be concluded that most of these thirty-three physicians became general officers on the basis of what they learned and did during the war itself.

The group of control generals contained more members who had prewar military training than did Group I. Six had graduated at West Point between 1833 and 1853 (Brooks, 1841; Chambers, 1853; Crook, 1852; Gardner, 1842; King, 1833; Michler, 1848). By 1861, all of them were still in the army except King. Page had been in the United States navy since 1824, advancing from midshipman to commander. He was an authority in ordnance and artillery and was used in this capacity by the Confederacy. Thirteen more had been trained variously in the state militias (nine), in the Mexican War (five), and in the Seminole War (one). The prior training is unknown in seven, and believed to have been nil in only six.

The information on the prior military training in the group of matching enlistees is less adequate than for the other groups. General George Sykes had graduated at West Point in 1842 and was a major by 1861. Gates had been in the New York militia. Granbury and Chapman had enlisted for the Mexican War, the latter as a private. Some others, no doubt, had military education, but the record of preparation appears even less impressive than that of the physician-generals.

No member of the matching surgeons group (Group IV) is known to have had a prior military education. Doctors Palmer and McGugin had been surgeons during the war in Mexico. It is said that Doctor George H. Lyman prepared before enlisting by assiduously studying about the medical department. He was rewarded by being promoted to the grade of medical inspector with the rank of lieutenant colonel, both unusual among the volunteers.

In looking at the 132 officers, then, fewer members of Group I has some form of military training than in Group II, but possibly more than in Group III, and definitely more than in Group IV. A number of the physician-generals, by having participated in military affairs, were not typical of American physicians of that time if the control surgeon group was representative of the medical profession.

Summary

In summary, it is evident that many members of the future physician-generals group before the war were already unusual in some respects but average in others in comparison with the control groups, especially the physicians of Group IV. They were typical of the time and profession in having been born in many different states of fathers representing many occupations, in having spent a predominantly rural boyhood, and in receiving a general education above average but only the usual two-year medical education or less. Many had migrated westward in accordance with the general movement of the times. They were atypical in that nine had already abandoned medicine before the war, and twenty-four had tried one or more occupations or professions in addition to medicine. Only ten seem to have been firmly committed to medicine. Chief among the additional occupations were law and politics. An unusually large number had travelled extensively for reasons other than for their medical education. More of them than of the control physicians had shown an interest in military affairs, but only one had received a military education, compared with six in the group of control generals.

Chapter V

WARTIME CAREERS

In this chapter the wartime records of the physician-generals are compared with those of the controls in a further search for evidence on why these doctors chose non-medical duty. Points of secondary interest were the reasons for their military success, and evidence that their men benefitted because they were physicians. Finally, figures were sought on the frequency and type of casualties in this sample group of 132 officers in which the count does not depend solely on the military records. In this sense it is a check on the completeness of those records.

Ranks and Grades Attained

Of the thirty-three physician-generals, six fought for the Confederacy and twenty-seven the Union. Of the latter, Myer was commissioned in only the regular army and Crawford in both the regular and the volunteer services. The others had commissions in either the volunteer Federal or the provisional Confederate armies. Eighteen were appointed general in the full grade—six Confederates and twelve Federals—and fifteen only by brevet. The numbers in the full grade were nearly proportional to the relative size of the two armies.

Eleven became major generals, but only three of them in the full rank (Anderson, Blunt, Leggett). Twenty-two were appointed brigadier general; nine of them had the full rank and thirteen only the brevet grade. The nine full brigadiers were Brandon, Bratton, Catterson, Gano, Kiernan, Myer, Northrop, Robertson, and Wild. Eight brigadiers were appointed additionally to be major generals by brevet; these were Bussey, Cameron, Capehart, Crawford, Harris, Kimball, McMillen and Scott. Generals Capehart and McMillen won no commission in the full grade but brevet appointments to both brigadier and major general. Crawford had the most awards in the rank of general: In the volunteers, he was commissioned a brigadier general in April, 1862 and a brevet major general in December, 1864, while in the regular army he was brevetted both brigadier and major general in March, 1865. Later, in 1875, he was retired as a full brigadier general, U.S.A. At least two generals holding brevet commissions were ordered assigned to duty in their brevet grade by the President—Leggett as a major general and Ludlow as a brigadier. Such presidential action was usually taken only when the military superior of the officer had so requested. A brevet commission did not automatically carry with it the military privileges and responsibilities of that grade.

The final rank achieved by the control generals by definition and selection equalled that of the physician-general they matched.

Promotion of the control physicians of Group IV was, in effect, limited by the nature of their commissions. They were unable to reach the high ranks attained by the physician-generals. Among the thousands of doctors who served in the medical departments as volunteers, only one reached general grade: Major Matthew McEwen, Surgeon of U. S. Volunteers, was awarded the rank of brigadier general by brevet at the end of the War *(Phisterer)*. As a Surgeon, U.S.V., he had already been higher in the power structure than a regimental surgeon. Medical officers in the volunteer service usually began as a regimental assistant surgeon with the equivalent rank usually of captain, or as a regimental surgeon (major). Eight doctors of Group IV were promoted from assistant surgeon to surgeon. Seventeen began as and remained surgeons even after long and faithful service. Three more had originally enlisted as privates (Anderson, Shepard, Speer) but were transferred and commissioned. Four were brevetted lieutenant colonel at the end of the war (Meeker, Norval, Smith, Speer). Doctors Duffee, Meeker, and Smith advanced from regimental to brigade surgeon by examination. Coolidge was promoted from surgeon to medical inspector (lieutenant colonel), both in the regular army. Among the volunteers, only Doctor Lyman went from brigade surgeon to medical inspector. Surgeon Samuel P. Moore left the United States Army and later became the confederate Surgeon-general, a position he filled creditably. His nominal equivalent grade of brigadier general seems not to have been actually conferred.

Considering that many of these doctors were beyond the usual military age and that their period of service was shortened by disease, they did well within the limits permitted by the army regulations. Some of them had already achieved medical distinction in civilian life before the war, and they were not rewarded proportionally to the physician-generals for their wartime contributions to the country.

The matching enlistees of Group III, unlike the control physicians, in theory had the same opportunity for advancement as did the future physician-generals, both groups originally enlisting in corresponding grades and positions. However, they fared far poorer on the average than the physician-generals group (see Table II). Their final ranks and the number of each were: one major general, three brigadier generals, eight brevet brigadier generals, six colonels, one brevet colonel, three lieutenant colonels, one major, four captains, one first lieutentant, and five surgeons. Thus, the group had only four general officers in the full grade and eight more by brevet. Five of these officers were never promoted even if they lost their lives in the army. These five include Colonel George T. Ward, killed at ten months; Captain Aldus J. Neff, dead of typhoid fever at fourteen months; Surgeon Thomas S. Neal, ineligible for promotion; and Lieutenant Colonel William E. Hadlock and Captain Louis F. Booth, who left the army at the expiration of their terms of enlistment, the latter after thirty-three months. It is clear that the physician-generals acquired more rank than their controls at enlistment

Although a number of the physician-generals used political influence, in accordance with their records of previous political activity in the statehouses, they were not regarded as "political generals" except for J. Patton Anderson and, possibly, Blunt, Bussey, and Wentworth. Crawford and others also used political influence although they were not professional politicians or known as political generals.

Length of Military Service

One possible factor that might influence the final rank is the length of military service. It was found that most of the physician-generals enlisted early. The average period of service was about forty-two months, calculated on the basis of a forty-eight month wartime maximum. Two (Crawford, Myer) had been in the army for some years, and three (Anderson, Bratton, Northrop) enlisted even before Fort Sumter fell. By the end of May, 1861, nineteen were already under arms. Of the remainder, all but three joined up in 1861. Only Champion, Harris, and Wentworth delayed enlisting till 1862. Only one (Elliott) served for less than a year and two others (Hillis, Wentworth) for less than two years. Elliott resigned under pressure, apparently unjustified, and Hillis and Wentworth had medical discharges.

The average length of service of the control generals was thirty-seven months, an average five months under that of the physician-generals. This is explained in part by less ardor for prompt enlistment and in part by more early deaths and discharges. Brigadier General Branch was killed at Antietam after seventeen months of service and Ellis at Gettysburg after eighteen months. Chickering left the army after twenty-two months with malaria and King at thirty months because of epilepsy. Generals Duryee, Lippitt, Williams, and Hillyer resigned for various reasons at seven, eighteen, nineteen, and twenty months, respectively. The career of six others possibly was impaired by capture and imprisonment: General George Crook was taken in bed, and five were taken in battle (Brevard, Leake, Miller, Michler, Page). As judged by the length of time needed to achieve general's stars, the performance of this group of officers was slightly better than that of the physician-generals. In part, this is explained by the seven who had received professional military educations.

The average length of service of the control enlistees, thirty-two months, was much less than that of the physician-generals. Only fifteen were in for forty months or longer. The average was reduced because the term of thirteen was shortened or terminated by death, disability, resignation, or discharge. Three were killed in battle (Black, Granbury, Ward), and three died of disease. Rutherford and Scott died of dysentery and Neff of typhoid fever. Cook, Gillespie, Hickcox, Pearce, Porter, and Willard were discharged for disability by disease, Rathbone was dismissed, and Neal resigned. With regard to death, disability, and shorter periods of service, the matching enlistee group represents better than the physician-generals group the average experience of the tens of thousands of the company and field grade officers in that war. It can, therefore, be argued that one factor in the achievement of general rank by some of the physician-generals was a long period of service made possible by serviceable health. At the time when they enlisted, the matching enlistees had the same chance for achieving distinction and advancement as the officers they matched. That they did not do so may be attributed to more fatal and nonfatal disease and to lesser abilities—military, political, and personal.

The control physicians averaged only thirty-three months of army service. Only fifteen were in for forty months or longer. Of the thirteen who served for thirty-two months or less, nine went home for disease, three for disability from wounds or injuries, and one for expiration of his nine-month term of enlistment. Medical discharges were the most numerous in this group. Whether this represents less endurance from older age, greater exposure to the infectious diseases in line of duty, or a lesser degree of fortitude is not known.

Thus, the physician-generals spent the longest average period in the army. The average time in months for the four groups was forty-two, thirty-seven, thirty-two, and thirty-three on the basis of a maximum of forty-eight months from April, 1861. This longer span is accounted for, in part, by fewer disabling wounds and diseases. The longer service, or the greater luck or vigor it represents may account, in part, for the reward of achieving higher ranks. The control generals won the same ranks slightly quicker but they had started with more military training.

Type of Military Service

The type of service assignment in part reflected ability, luck, and influence, and it might influence promotions. The physician-generals of Group I filled a wide range of positions during the war. Thirty of them led combat troops in the field at one time or another. Doctor Elwell had only quartermaster duty and Northrop was the commissary-general at Richmond. Myer, as the chief signal officer, organized the newly created signal corps in the grade of colonel for some months before the appointment lapsed through the opposition of Secretary Stanton. By then, he had trained other members of the signal service. Crawford went directly from the staff to a brigade command, but all of the other twenty-nine field officers at one time led regiments. Twenty-four of them eventually had brigades as well, thirteen led divisions, and three (Cameron, Crawford, and Leggett) temporarily directed army corps. Finally, Blunt commanded an army —the Army of the Frontier—for some months. At least ten had experience in staff positions. Blunt had charge of a military department, and six managed districts of various sizes and importance at one time or another. Of those who led troops, twenty-four had infantry, three led cavalry, and two had both. Brown and Kiernan commanded only negro troops. Blunt headed Indian, Negro and white soldiers at one time. Brandon and Northrop had bureau jobs for a while. After the war a number stayed on in the Freedman's Bureau. These various assignments indicate a wide range of talent in leadership and administration.

Among the control generals, the type of service was essentially like that of the physician-generals; their ranks were matching by definition and selection. Their commands were infantry (twenty-five), cavalry (two), and both (two). Attorney Hillyer had only staff duty with Grant and Lawyer Kinsman with General Butler. Michler's service was limited to engineering and Page's to ordnance, engineering, and coast artillery. Major General John Logan, as one of the ablest political generals, commanded the Army of the Tennessee, temporarily during the battle of Atlanta and permanently at war's end. Generals Brooks, Crook, and Logan led army corps. Generals Bate, Caldwell, Carr, and King had divisions. The others led brigades or regiments. Welsh had only a regiment of colored infantry. Brooks directed the Department of the Monongahela at Pittsburg in 1863 during Lee's invasion of Pennsylvania. Six had district or subdistrict commands at one time or another: Byrne and Chickering headed districts in Louisiana under Banks, Crook was in West Virginia, Gardner in Florida, Lippitt in northern California, and McNeil in Missouri.

Original Rank

The thirty-three doctors in Group I became generals from unimpressive beginnings. At least four of them (Blunt, Bratton, Catterson,

Zulich) had enlisted as privates, but most of them had already been promoted in camp before they were mustered into the Federal or Confederate services. Five had begun as surgeons or assistant surgeons (Brown, Capehart, Crawford, Kiernan, McMillen). Four had duty as aides to governors or a general before receiving commissions with regiments (Bussey, Hillis, Leggett, Wentworth). The governors could give little military education but they wielded political power in making appointments and promotions. One began as an assistant quartermaster with the rank of captain. The remaining twenty started with troops: One began as a lieutenant, ten as captains, three as majors, five as lieutenant colonels, and only one (Anderson) as a colonel. In four years or less, they reached the general ranks already described.

The matching enlistees, by definition, had the same first ranks. Most of the physicians in the medical department (Group IV) began as assistant surgeons or as surgeons. The future generals in Group II originally held ranks ranging from private (Bate, Branch, Duryee, Hillyer, Welsh, Zinn) to brigadier general in the case of Rufus King, an ex-officer of the army (see Table I). Ten began as colonels and ten as captains. Confederate Brigadier General Richard L. Page had been a commander in the U. S. Navy.

Age at Enlistment

When the war began the future physician-generals averaged 36.9 years of age. The range was from twenty-three to fifty-seven years. Nineteen were age thirty-five or older, and five were over forty-five years. Some were above the draft age, and many were in the age in which men tended to do poorly under strenuous field life. Knowing that these officers were physicians, it is safe to maintain that this age structure reflects maturity and experience of sorts. At the same time it is obvious that the physicians who chose combat duty were not young hot-heads.

The physician-generals were very slightly older than the control generals of Group II, whose average age was 34.5 years, with a range of nineteen to fifty-three. The matching enlistees of Group III averaged 34.7 years of age, with a range of twenty-two to fifty-six. The control surgeons (Group IV) were the oldest. They averaged

40.2 years and the range was from twenty-four to fifty-four years. The age is known for only thirty members of this group, of whom twenty were thirty-five years or older and eleven were over age forty-five. It is apparent that as far as the physicians were concerned this was not a young man's war, and it was broadly supported. It is seen that the average age of the physician-generals was nearly the same as that of the control generals and the matching enlistees, all of which were lower than that of the control physicians. The average age of these four officer groups was far above that of the enlisted men. The mean age of 303,148 enlistees was 27.3 years *(Baxter)*.

Probably, the only group of soldiers older than such officer groups was the "Gray-Beard Regiment"—the Iowa Thirty-seventh Volunteers. This was a regiment especially authorized by Secretary Stanton for limited duty, in which every member was over age forty-five and thus draft-proof *(Ingersoll)*. It was mustered in at Muscatine in December, 1862 and served until May, 1865 in guarding railroads and military prisons, and on picket duty in Iowa, Tennessee, and Ohio. From colonel to drummer boy every member was over forty-five and one private claimed he was over eighty. It had two men killed and two wounded in action.

The age characteristics yield no clue why some physicians chose combat duty.

Date of the Generalcy

Although a few of these physicians became generals quickly, most of them needed three or four years to acquire this rank. None were so promoted in 1861, but Anderson, Blunt, Crawford, Kimball, Leggett, and Robertson were general officers by the end of 1862, three more in 1863, and seven in 1864. Fifteen were first appointed in this rank after the war to date from March, 1865 or later. Myer was belatedly promoted in 1866 for his war services and his commission was dated back to March, 1865.

The members of Group II were, on the whole, advanced to general no faster than the physicians, except that four were so promoted already in 1861. Three of the four were West Point graduates (Brooks, Gardner, King) and one (Branch) was a politician with little military training. Among the remainder, seven first became generals in 1862, three in 1863, two in 1864, and the final seventeen in 1865.

The promotion of the eleven matching enlistees who won general rank was at about the same rate as in Groups I and II; one in 1861, one in 1862, three in 1864, and six in 1865.

In summary, as judged by the speed with which they were promoted to the rank of general, the physician-generals did neither better nor worse than those control generals who had similar military backgrounds.

Duty as General Officers Prior to the Appointment

Although some of the officers of Group I had never carried out the duties of a general officer before their promotion, most of them had served in the higher position, some of them for a long time. Thus, Capehart, Catterson, Champion, Dustin, Leasure, and Miller had commanded brigades for periods varying from five to twenty-four months, and Dustin and Leasure had the occasional temporary responsibility even for divisions before they were awarded their stars. Among those promoted to general at the end of the war, Brown, Elliott, Elwell, Lippincott, Myer, and Zulich had not acted in the capacity of generals according to the records. The same statement is true of Hillis, Wainwright, and Wentworth, but these three officers had resigned in 1863 or 1864 for disability. Many other disabled field grade officers were rewarded by a promotion in 1865.

The record of the control generals of Group II is essentially like that of Group I. On the whole, there appears in both groups to have been more undue leniency in awarding the general grade to some questionably deserving it than for withholding the rank from the deserving. An outstanding example of apparent injustice is the case of Alexander Chambers. This professionally educated officer as a lieutenant mustered in fourteen Iowa regiments in 1861 before accepting the colonelcy of a new regiment for himself. He did well, led brigades, was wounded in battle three times, and was appointed a brigadier in 1863. However, the senate failed to confirm, and the commission had to be revoked in 1864, so he reverted to the rank of captain in the regular army. The confirmation failed because no politicians would accept him as a general on their informal state quota. He had been appointed to West Point from New York but his father later moved to Minnesota and Chambers gave that state as his residence in 1861. Neither Iowa, New York, or Minnesota would support or credit him to its quota in 1863. He died in 1888 at age fifty-four, having suffered at times from his wounds, without having been rewarded in proportion to many less deserving.

As judged by their previous duty assignments, most of the physician-generals deserved their stars fully as much as the control generals.

Service with Negro Troops or in the Freedman's Bureau

A relatively high proportion (nearly one-third) of these doctors at one time commanded Negro troops or served in the Freedman's Bureau. Doctors Brown and Wild did both. Harris and Scott were in the Freedman's service after the war. Doctors Blunt, Cameron, Catterson, Kiernan, Ludlow, McMillen, and Wild led colored regiments or brigades. Of this group Wild seems to have done the best by recruiting and training "Wild's African Brigade" in Virginia and North Carolina in 1864. None of these troops won any striking successes but they were not all tested in combat. As in the example of Wild and several others, it seems that these ex-physicians were dedicated to this type of service. In other cases, this duty may have been chosen to gain personal advancement. As general officers, none of these men can be regarded as outstanding beyond question, and the competence in this grade of several is questionable.

Far fewer of the control generals served with Negroes. Two (Carr, Welsh) led colored troops late in the war, but none worked in the Freedman's Bureau afterward, although Kinsman, as a staff officer with Butler, had earlier been concerned with Negro affairs in occupied territory in the Department of the Gulf. Among the matching enlistees of Group III, only Gates had duty with Negro organizations. The control surgeons, by the nature of their enlistments and selection had no service with Negro regiments.

It is apparent, then, that a higher proportion of the physician-generals than of the officers in the control Groups II and III served with Negro troops or in the Freedman's Bureau. To what extent this signifies either special interest or personal ambition is not known.

Role of Wounds and Disease

Sickness and disease played a big role in the military careers of the physician-generals and the controls just as they did for all soldiers. Among the one hundred and thirty-two officers, nine died during the war—five in battle and four of camp diseases. None of the nine were physician-generals but six were matching enlistees, two were control generals, and one was a control physician. Generals Branch and Ellis of Group II died of wounds in battle. Surgeon Gans of Group IV died of an unnamed acute camp infection. In Group III, Black, Granbury, and Ward died of wounds, Rutherford and Scott of dysentery, and Neff of typhoid fever.

Medical discharges were given during the war to four members of Group I (Hillis, Kiernan, Wainwright, Wentworth), to four of Group II (Brooks, Hillyer, King, Sewell), to five in Group III (Cook, Hickcox, Pearce, Porter, Willard), and to at least eleven of the surgeons in Group IV (Allen, Duffee, Harrison, Hurd, Martin, McGugin, McPheeters, Newhaus, Salter, Smith, Udell). Of the twenty-four medical discharges, four were for wounds and twenty for disease. Group III suffered most severely from death and discharge, and Group IV lost the most members from discharge for disease.

The total number of casualties was large for each group. The figures are found in Table IV. The one hundred and thirty-two members of the four groups together suffered ninety-seven known wounds and injuries and 128 recorded attacks of disease, for a total of 225 diagnoses. These figures are short of actuality, and they are most nearly complete for the doctors in Groups I and IV.

The physician-generals suffered severely. In April, 1861, many were in the older age groups and many of them spent most of the

TABLE IV

COMPARISON OF THE NUMBER OF CASUALTIES IN THE FOUR GROUPS

	Physician-generals	*Control Generals*	*Matching Enlistees*	*Control Physicians*	*All Groups*
Wounds and injuries	43	30	17	7	97
Diseases	36	29	32	31	128
Totals	79	59	49	38	225

war as officers of field grade, in whom combat and camp casualties were high. No medical history has been found for Myer or Northrop and the record is incomplete on many others. Being physicians, many of these officers treated themselves off the record when ill. As high ranking officers, they had special care when wounded and some wounds did not get into the records. However, the incomplete record reveals forty-three wounds and injuries and thirty-six illnesses, an average of about two and one-half for each officer in the group.

The diseases include nine cases of dysentery or diarrhea, four each of malaria, rheumatism and hemorrhoids, two of bronchitis, two of unspecified chest diseases probably tuberculosis, one each of cystitis, jaundice, acute purulent ophthalmia, yellow fever, boils, bilious fever, heart disease, and erysipelas, and three unidentified "fevers." Hemorrhoids were regarded as a medical disease at that time and often as following prolonged diarrhea. Some of these diseases recurred once or more times, resulting in much loss of time. It is probable that this list is far short of reality. For example, the reported cases of diarrhea and dysentery in the Union army alone numbered about 1,700,000—about two for each three men. Nine examples of this disease in the thirty-three officers is far short of their expected quota.

The record of wounds is also impressive. Fourteen wounds were not further described. There were at least fifteen gunshot and one shrapnel wound, resulting in the amputation of one arm and one leg. Fourteen traumatic injuries of various types included two ventral hernias, three leg fractures, one concussion, one penetrating abdominal wound, and a number of other inadequately documented injuries.

There is little evidence that these medical and surgical conditions greatly influenced the careers of these officers, except that disease terminated the service of three and wounds of one. The diseases, if prolonged, might have delayed promotions. Wounds, in contrast, as a mark of valor in battle, were likely to aid advancement. Only Wentworth's army life was cut short by a wound.

Such records as exist for the control generals are not all complete. Nevertheless, seventeen of them had a total of twenty-seven wounds and three injuries. Two wounds, both head shots, were fatal (Branch, Ellis). Twenty-six of the wounds were caused by bullets and one by a shell. This fact shows that these officers were up at the immediate line of impact. The injuries were usually caused by shot horses or the nearby explosion of shells. Four officers in the group had three wounds apiece (Bate, Chambers, Sewell, and Zinn). In sixteen of the control generals, no record of wounding or injury has been found.

Among the matching enlistees, histories of wounds are lacking in sixteen, of disease in eight, and of both in three. Seventeen members of the group suffered seventeen wounds or injuries, three of which were fatal (Black, Granbury, Ward). Four gunshot, one shell, one bayonet, and one wound of unstated cause were recorded. Of the eight injuries, six were caused by horses. Horses sometimes fell or became unmanageable when shot; others became unruly when frightened by explosions.

Thirty-two illnesses occurred among twenty-five officers in Group III. Eight had dysentery or diarrhea, from which two died during the war and others suffered after returning home. Four had typhoid fever, from which one died. Other diseases, represented by one example each, were smallpox, tuberculosis, granular ophthalmia, pleuritis, jaundice, scurvy, sunstroke, biliary fever, and inflammatory rheumatism. Piles accounted for two victims, and in nine the precise diagnosis has not been found.

The control surgeons reported as many illnesses and injuries as the members of the other groups, but fewer wounds. Twelve left no account of any disease, but the other twenty-one suffered thirty-one illnesses. Dysentery or diarrhea was the commonest diagnosis, with eight cases. The others were malaria (three), tuberculosis (three), rheumatism (two), hemorrhoids (two), and one case each of typhoid fever, typho-malaria, neuralgia, jaundice, asthma, bronchitis, and hepatitis. For six illnesses, no diagnosis has been found. Of the three physicians with cough and hemoptysis that led to a diagnosis of tuberculosis and to medical discharge, all survived the war for many years, two reaching the ages of eighty-five and seventy-four years. The prognosis of pulmonary tuberculosis was not invariably bad as was sometimes supposed.

The control physicians received far fewer combat wounds than the members of the other groups as would be expected. Five surgeons suffered a total of seven traumatic casualties. Four were injured, one developed an erysipelas after operating on an infected wound, and one was twice wounded. Surgeon Newhaus was shot at Winchester early in 1862. On August 29, 1862, in the battle of Second Bull Run, he was again shot while dressing wounded men on the battlefield. The clavicle and the acromial process of the scapula were fractured, and he was pensioned for permanent disability. He died in 1866, but the relation of death to the wound was not a matter of record *(Newhaus)*.

In conclusion, the casualties were high in all four groups. Slightly more illnesses and wounds plus injuries were found for the physician-generals than for the members of the other three groups (see Table IV). The records, however, in Group I are better than for the other groups, and it is believed that the actual frequency was about proportional to the length of time served and that the differences are not significant except for fewer wounds among the control physicians. The physician-generals were not exceptionally valorous, and their achievement of the rank of general cannot be ascribed as a reward for an undue number of casualties in combat.

Promotion Despite Disability

Many officers were promoted to general rank in the Civil War despite having a physical disability. Some were totally incapacitated at the time, but others were able to hold administrative positions in rear areas, and a few were permitted to return to field duty with some degree of disability. Generals John B. Hood, Richard Ewell, Oliver O. Howard, and Philip Kearny were a few of the many generals permitted to take the field after amputations in a day when that duty required the ability to manage fractious horses. Here, we are ignoring the many officers who were promoted while suffering from chronic dysentery, tuberculosis, malaria and other diseases from which they were periodically disabled. Neither are we here concerned with the many awards to general grade, often by brevet, as a deliberate reward for disabling wounds. Most of these were conferred after the war but pre-dated. Some examples of such reward of disability are Generals Elwell, Hillis, and Wainwright in Group I and Chickering and Hillyer in Group II.

In Group I, other examples of promotion despite a disability are

Doctor Kiernan, who was made a brigadier general in August, 1863, although he then had an incompletely healed chest shot wound, from which he was incapacitated and discharged a few months later. Wild was commissioned a brigadier in April, 1863, although his left arm had been amputated near the shoulder and the first and second fingers of his right hand were permanantly stiffened. He was permitted to return to active duty, at times with cavalry. Brandon lost a leg in 1862. In 1864, he was promoted to brigadier general and assigned to a recruiting position in Mississippi, for which he was eminently fitted by his knowledge, prestige, age, and battle scar. Gano was commissioned a general and permitted to remain in the field with cavalry despite the impaired use of an arm.

In Group II, Bate remained in the field and was promoted successively to brigadier and major general although he had a stiffened knee from a wound at Shiloh. Under similar circumstances, Gardner was also retained in service and given limited duty assignments. Brooks was made a general although his health had been poor for many years because of a urethral stricture. His war service was impaired by the same lesion, from the effects of which he died in 1870. Brigadier General Rufus King broke down with epilepsy at the battle of Second Bull Run while holding a divisional command, and he died from the progression of this disease a few years later. If this disease existed prior to enlistment, he should not have been commissioned and placed under this additional stress; if it came on in the service, he should later have been awarded a major generalcy by brevet.

Promotion of the disabled sometimes filled vacant commissions that were badly needed for the advancement of others. An even greater problem was created by promoting disabled and then assigning them duties for which they were now physically or mentally disqualified, unfitted, or inefficient. Often, the surgeons either were not asked for an opinion in the matter or, if consulted, they were unable in many cases to give sound advice. Any adverse military consequences resulting from such unsuited assignments of the members of these groups are hard to detect because these officers did not hold important large and stressful positions. Bad effects can be recognized, however, in the experiences of others such as Ewell, A. P. Hill *(Steiner)* and many others.

Evidence of a Prior Medical Education

Here, interest centers on whether there was any evidence from their wartime actions or the records of their commands that these officers had a medical education. Were the health records of their commands better than those of others? Did they have fewer medical discharges for conditions that had existed prior to enlistment or for camp diseases? Was the mortality in their men from wounds lower because of better hemostasis on the battlefields, better collection and transportation to the rear, or better treatment in the regimental and brigade hospitals? Were their men better fed to avoid scurvy? Were they better protected against the elements in the winter camps? Did their medical officers receive exceptional support in matters of camp sanitation, medical supplies and facilities, and evacuation of the sick and wounded?

All of these questions must be answered in the negative. In fact, only Doctor Leasure left any evidence that he was a physician: He helped his surgeons operate after battle and he once criticised the medical supply situation. The others, including the five who began the war as medical officers, left no indications of a prior medical education except for the occasional use of medical terms by Crawford. Men in the regiment of ex-doctor Leggett developed smallpox, although vaccination was available and its use encouraged if not required. He could have pressured his surgeon to vaccinate. Champion's men had scurvy during the winter of 1863-64 and much camp disease. Miller's regiment left behind it the trail of death from disease described in his biography. A few complimented their surgeons in post-action reports, but there is no evidence that their men had better surgical care than those in other commands. General Crawford had ten years of experience in military medicine before the war but his numerous regiments (about forty-one) were not kept healthier than others, and he had to be chided for negligence in draining his campsite as late as 1864 when malaria was highly prevalent. Some of the regimental histories fail even to mention that the colonel had been a physician; although the historians must have been aware of this fact, they did not think it important.

This situation shows as well as any other the undeveloped state of medical knowledge as well as failure to use the available knowledge. Unless it is claimed that these thirty-three doctors were all incompetent, vicious, not conscientious, or exceptionally ignorant, it must be concluded that this record reflects a general ignorance or indifference.

Inasmuch as the control surgeons were in the same regiments as the future physician-generals, they must share with the latter the blame for this record, if blame is due. Since the control surgeon group included many physicians who were able if not superior, according to their pre- and postwar records, this state of affairs in military medicine must reflect, in part, the various inadequacies of the times.

Reason for Choosing the Fighting Services

As far as is known, none of the thirty-three physician-generals left an explanation of why he abandoned the scalpel for the sword. An officer with Crawford at Fort Sumter wrote that he was ambitious for military distinction but he gave no evidence *(Doubleday)*. Of Capehart it was said that the preferred fighting to healing. Jefferson Davis probably had little difficulty convincing Doctor Northrop, an old friend and former army officer now doctoring the Negroes in Charleston, that an important future awaited him as commissary-general. Many of these doctors enlisted as early as April (twelve) or May (three) of 1861. They had little time in which to close out their medical practice. It seemed that the war would be short. To grab a gun and rush off to lick the enemy was almost as natural as it had been in the Revolution. One must look into other aspects of their record to discover why these doctors chose combat commissions. This will be done in Chapter VII.

Military Efficiency and Distinction

The military efficiency, capacity, and contributions of some of these physicians are evaluated with difficulty because they were not fully developed. Some were handicapped or lost time on account of wounds or illness. Others had unlucky assignments or made a late start and were still rising at the end. However, as judged principally from the *Official Records* the greatest military distinction in the group was achieved by Doctors Anderson, Crawford, Kimball, and Leggett. Perhaps Blunt should be added to this group. His military record is hard to judge in comparison with that of the others because it all took place in the West beyond the main stream of the war effort. Northrop served only as a commissary-general and Brown and Elwell as assistant quartermasters, both positions in which the achievement of military distinction was difficult. Northrop won prominence but of an unfortunate type. The commanders of regiments and brigades had little opportunity to win distinction except in battles, but battles were usually far apart and a few officers were never in combat. Only Anderson, Crawford, and Leggett advanced to divisional commands and remained there under the stiff, grinding demands of a major army. However, Bratton, Harris, McMillen, Miller, and several others were still on the upgrade under those conditions in 1865. Myer did well with developing the signal service but had the misfortune to antagonize Secretary Stanton. Kimball performed important political chores for President Lincoln on two occasions, and Harris became a member of the court trying the assassination conspirators. Several did not do well under army discipline and came before military courts (Robertson, Wild). Doctors Capehart and Wentworth were awarded the Medal of Honor. Of the thirty-three, only nineteen served during the war years while holding the rank of general.

The control generals, selected because they matched the physician-generals in final rank, were militarily not more outstanding even if the six having a professional education (Brooks, Chambers, Crook, Gardner, King, Michler,) are included. Of these West Point graduates, Brooks and Crook were the most successful, but they did not achieve conspicuous success, and Brooks resigned in 1864. His name had been included by Burnside after the battle of Fredericksburg among those he wished dismissed from the army—recommendations not approved by the President. Among the volunteers Logan stood out throughout the war, especially at Fort Donelson, Vicksburg, and in Georgia. Hartranft was on a sharp upgrade at the end, while Caldwell and Carr were on the downgrade. Some of the others also were improving with experience. Only sixteen members of the group had duty while in general grade, but two others performed the services of a general although not holding the rank.

Among the twelve generals in the group of matching enlistees, only Sykes and Gorgas were prominent. Gorgas did an outstanding job in organizing and operating an ordnance department for the South, although his past record had not revealed this potential. Sykes regressed after 1863 and was sent to the west. From military grades originally the same as those of their physician-general counterparts, the other thirty-one matching enlistees did not reach corresponding distinction.

A certain degree of correlation is found between the military distinction achieved and the amount of prior military training. This relationship is evident in both Groups I and II. The data are inadequate to show whether this is a cause-and-effect relationship or whether the prior participation in military affairs merely indicates exceptional interest and native ability.

Crossing of Paths During the War

The number of physician-generals was large enough so that on the basis of chance some paths should have crossed. This is found actually to have occurred many times. Yet there is no evidence of mutual recognition of the previous physician status. Some fought against each other, some served together, and some were subordinates of others. They met in rear districts as well as in all of the main armies—the Armies of the Tennessee, Cumberland, Potomac, James, and others.

The largest number was concentrated under Grant at Vicksburg. Here were collected Doctors Bussy, Cameron, Hillis, Hillyer, Kiernan, Kimball, Leasure, Leggett, Lippincott, McMillen, and Scott. Grant's forces in the west always had a high proportion of the non-professional, volunteer officers, and the greater part of five army corps were concentrated here before the siege ended. A part of Grant's genius consisted of developing such officers.

The next largest number was found in the army group of Sherman (Armies of the Ohio, Cumberland, Tennessee, and Georgia) in the Atlanta, Savannah, and Carolina campaigns. On duty here were Catterson, Champion, Dustin, Kimball, Leggett, Miller, Scott and Zulich, while Anderson was in the opposing army. In the Army of the Potomac, at one time or another were Doctors Crawford, Kimball, Leasure, Wainwright, and Zulich while in the opposing

Army of Northern Virginia, Bratton and Robertson were defending Northrop in nearby Richmond. In the adjacent Army of the James were Harris, Ludlow, and Wild. At about the same time in Arkansas and the Indian Territory Gano and Robertson were opposed by Blunt and Kimball. In 1861, Doctors Crawford, Harris, Kimball, Miller and others were involved in the tedious operations in West Virginia launched earlier by McClellan, with whom Leggett had served. Kiernan and Ludlow were in General Fremont's strange cavalry entourage around St. Louis at that time. Others converged in the Department of the Gulf, at Mobile in 1865, and elsewhere. It is regrettable that they did not organize yet another special society.

Original Medical and Military Contributions

Lessons from the Civil War applicable to military medicine and surgery today are few. The upsurge in scientific medicine later in the century outmoded most of what had been learned between 1861 and 1865. Some of the lessons learned in microbiology after 1880 were not fully applied even during the Spanish-American war, and the typhoid fever and dysentery of that war were in large part inexcusable. By World War I, military medicine was able to bring a new ratio to combat casualties in relation to medical disease. And by World War II, preventive immunizations, atabrine, DDT, mobile shower baths and clothes sterilizers, packaged food, blood and plasma, chlorinated water, penicillin, diesel fuel, bulldozers and other improved methods of field sanitation had made most of the lessons of the Civil War obsolete except that of the need for alertness and the will to learn and change.

One ex-Confederate surgeon, on the basis of a vast personal experience with 12,000 patients seen in field and general hospitals, in 1874 summarized the lessons learned *(Satchwell):* Many doctors had become proficient in the use of chloroform, and they had learned much about the natural course of wounds and disease. For example, consumption sometimes improved on field service, children from poor scrofulous parents did better than those from mansions, and tents were better than elegant closed structures for men with erysipelas, typho-malaria, gangrene, and some other diseases. In surgery, they learned that bones sometimes reproduced from a vestige of periosteum, bullet forceps were useless, primary hemorrhage on the field could be disregarded, and few types of surgical wounds and injuries were invariably fatal. The limited value of these bits of information today is obvious.

None of the thirty-three physician-generals made any original and new contribution to military science. It can be argued that some of them might have left more to posterity if they had been in the medical service. This possibility was unpredictable and probably did not occur to them. Of the nine who were with Sherman in Georgia and the Carolinas, none performed a military service that could not have been done equally well by others, and none left much for the record. In contrast, one of Sherman's physicians, Surgeon Edmund Andrews of Chicago, in 1866 published a vivid account of the campaign with emphasis on the primary surgery on the 6,122 wounded *(Andrews and Woodworth)*. From this vast experience they learned that nearly all wounded men did well when transported in ambulances in the open (i.e., wagons); they did not have to be abandoned when an army was on the move. This lesson learned from the first use of large scale mobile warfare has subsequently had little application, even in the recent mobile warfare, and it seems to have played no part in the discovery of the value of early ambulation.

Like the members of the control groups, these physician-generals made no original contributions to either military or to medical science. But in a time of great national stress they practiced reasonably well the known, and nearly all of them faithfully performed their duty to the best of their abilities. They shared the hardships and risks with their men, asking no favors. They earned the gratitude of the nation.

Chapter VI

POSTWAR LIFE

FURTHER ATTEMPTS TO account for the main phenomenon under study are made in this chapter. The postwar careers are especially informative on the strength of the interest of these doctors in medicine.

Date of Discharge

The troops were rapidly discharged after the war which, in the southwest ended only in May, 1865. The Confederate soldiers were free to go home as soon as they had been paroled. The mustering out of the Union soldiers began soon after the big Victory parades in Washington on May 23rd and 24th. Most of the men in the eleven army corps concentrated in the east were home by the end of August, as were most of the other troops. A few units were held in the South or sent to Texas.

The general officers did not get out quite so fast. By April 15, 1865, twenty-six members of Group I had already served for forty months or longer, and many of them were able to leave that year. Generals Catterson, Elwell, and Harris went home only in 1866. Brown and Scott remained in the Freedman's Bureau until 1868. Crawford stayed in the army until 1873 and Myer until his death in 1880. In Group II, five members remained in the army: Generals Byrne, Chambers, Crook, Michler, and Welsh had to take lower ranks in the regular army but they stayed on. Eleven others were already out before the end of 1864 because of death, disability, resignation, or expiration of their term of enlistment. Eight were discharged in 1865 and four in 1866. Thus, fewer members of Group I showed continuing military interest than of Group II.

Residual Disease and Disability

The life of many of these physician-generals was permanently changed by the war. Some were never again well. Many went home with residual diseases or disabilities that shortened their lives, influenced their careers, or made existence miserable. The same statement can be made for the officers in the other groups. The record is far from complete, but of the one hundred and twenty-four surviving officers in the four groups, sixty-nine went home with some degree of disability. Their pathological diagnoses totalled eighty-eight, inasmuch as some had more than one. Of the eighty-eight diagnoses, fifty-eight were medical and thirty resulted from wounds or injuries. The commonest residual diseases were chronic dysentery or diarrhea (eleven cases), rheumatism (nine examples), malaria (eight), hemorrhoids, often following diarrhea in horseback riders (seven), and tuberculosis and other chronic lung disorders (eleven). The commonest post-traumatic residual was a bad leg with lameness from wounds and various other causes, present in nine officers, old back injuries (four), stiffened fingers and hands (three), and the post-concussion effects from shell explosions (three), or falls from horses. Some of these partly disabled men had gone home during the war but others hung on to the end.

The members of Groups I and IV recorded the most residuals. Whether this actually represents more disease or whether, being physicians, they knew the pension advantage of having abnormalities mentioned in their record, must remain uncertain.

Four members of Group I left the army during the war: Hillis resigned in 1863 for rheumatism, Wainwright in 1863 for malaria and a chest disease, Kiernan in 1864 for malaria and a thoracic wound, and Wentworth left in 1864 for a gunshot wound through the body. All continued to suffer after the war.

Ten additional physician-generals went home after the war with some degree of disability from wounds. Brandon had lost a leg and Wild an arm. Wild had also two stiffened fingers in his remaining hand. Crawford, Elwell, Leasure, and Miller had crippling effects from old leg wounds and Miller also suffered from an old cerebral concussion. McMillen had two stiffened fingers and Gano an arm. Leggett carried a traumatic umbilical hernia, and Scott injuries of the back and knee. In addition, thirteen on discharge had residual service-incurred disease of the types already mentioned.

At least four physician-generals had greatly shortened lives. Kiernan died in 1869 at age thirty-two years of malaria and disease of the lungs that produced an occasional hemoptysis. Champion died in 1873 at age forty-seven of consumption. Zulich died in 1876, aged fifty-two years, with a chronic diarrhea and "cheesy deposits" not located but said to result from the wartime enteritis. Blunt died in 1881 of a cerebral disorder that began in 1863. The deaths of several others were regarded as service-related by the pension bureau. The pathetic account of Doctor Capehart's moving from hilly to level country for heart disease so that he could continue to practice, by carriage rather than on horseback, has already been related.

Medical Training from the War Experience

In view of the large experience with wounds and disease during the war, especially by the five who had served for a while as medical officers, did these physician-generals and the control physicians profit professionally by this medical experinece? No evidence is found that they did. On the contrary, many of them lost ground professionally. They made no medical discoveries or advances. No great surgical advances and few minor improvements that they could have learned and adopted from others came from the vast war experience. The management of penetrating wounds of the head, thorax, abdomen, and pelvis was not greatly improved. In the treatment of wounds of the extremities, the question of conservative versus radical management was not settled; the indication for excisions as against amputations also was not clarified. Wound infections, shock, primary and secondary hemorrhage, and bed sores existed in 1865 as before. Unquestionably, some doctors had learned skillfully to administer chloroform and ether anesthesia, and many had acquired technical skill in traumatic surgery which would be of some but limited use in general practice. Little progress had been made in the prevention, improved diagnosis, or better treatment of the acute infectious diseases or others. It is true that a little progress was made in understanding the course of some diseases in special studies set up in rear area hospitals by a few physicians such as S. Weir Mitchell in Philadelphia. However, no great immediate practical advances came from such investigations.

Inasmuch as fewer physicians of Group I returned to the practice of medicine after 1865 than had left it in 1861, collectively they lost ground professionally by the war. The medically most successful members of the group—Hillis and Leasure—were successful for reasons other than their war experience. Doctor Leasure was successful already before the war, and Hillis specialized in the diseases of women and children. The same statements can be made for the five physicians among the matching enlistees.

The influence of their war experience on the professional capabilities of the members of Group IV is harder to judge. Doctors Duffee, Jones, Lyman, Meeker, Newman, Palmer, D. P. Smith, and Speer seem to have been exceptionally successful. In every instance, however, they were successful already before the war or they became prominent in a field not especially related to their war experience. Possibly, some others among the twenty-one in practice became better physicians as a result of their army service in ways that are not apparent. This is unlikely because of the nature of the advances coming from the war. The improvements in military medicine between 1861 and 1865 came principally in the form of better organization, administration, and supply (i.e., in the mechanics of medical care) rather than from scientific advances in the knowledge, diagnosis, and treatment of wounds and disease.

Return to the Practice of Medicine and Teaching

The war had cost most of the physicians of Group I up to four years of their life by April, 1865. A number of them still suffered from impaired health. They averaged nearly forty-one years of age. As before the war, their interests were numerous and scattered. Only six returned to the practice of medicine for a while, eight more practiced occasionally or part time, but nineteen never practiced again. Of the six who practiced full time, three did well: Doctor Leasure had a large practice and he published some excellent clinical studies. Hillis, out of practice in 1861, now took postgraduate studies and specialized in the diseases of women and children. He was also long connected with the Keokuk College of Physicians and Surgeons. Elliott resumed the practice of ophthalmology in New York City. Brown, Cameron, and Blunt were also successful. Among the eight who practiced occasionally or briefly, Capehart, Kiernan, Ludlow, and Miller were in poor health, while Doctors Dustin, Harris, Wentworth, and Robertson had divided interests, all mixing in local or state politics.

The postwar medical interest of the control physician group was, quantitatively and qualitatively, far greater than that of the physician-generals. Twenty-one returned to the practice or teaching of medicine as their vocation and eight more had a part time practice. One died during the war (Gans) and another at its end (McGugin), both of disease contracted in line of duty. The postwar fate of the remaining two (Norval, Shepard) is unknown. Nearly all of the part time practitioners were such because of service-incurred disability. Some of the full time doctors also were handicapped by partial disability resulting from their war experiences. Nevertheless, some of them were exceptionally successful. One must conclude that the medical interest, if not also competence, of the physician-generals was far inferior to that of the control physicians after the war.

The five physicians in Group III are too few for statistical analyses, but their postwar experience seems to have resembled that of the physician-generals more than the control physician group. Doctor McDermont returned to a successful practice in Dayton, and Brown was on duty in the army medical service until his death from tuberculosis in 1889. In the interim, he had published some nice studies. Doctors Herrick, Neal, and Willard suffered from disease contracted in the army; Herrick died from chronic diarrhea in 1873 and Willard from consumption in 1870.

As far as is known, the physician-generals took little interest in medical organizations or education except for Hillis, who taught at the College of Physicians and Surgeons at Keokuk, Iowa, and for Elwell, who taught legal medicine in several medical and law schools in the Cleveland area. Doctors Kiernan and McMillen did not return to medical editing after the war. Doctor Brown was the President of the Connecticut Medical Society in 1889.

Many of the control physicians, in contrast, were interested in medical organizations, schools, and authorship. Doctor Thomas M. Palmer, as the president of the Florida Medical Association from 1876 to 1878, delivered his presidential address on the early history of medicine in that state *(Palmer)*. Doctor David P. Smith held membership in the American Medical Association, the American Public Health Association, the Massachusetts Medical Society, and other professional organizations. Doctor David McGugin became the President of the Iowa State Medical Society and other groups. Doctor George H. Lyman was the President of the Massachusetts Medical Society, a founder of the American Gynecological Society, and was interested in other organizations. Doctor Milhau was a member of the American Public Health Association, the New York Pathological Society, and other groups. Other members of the American Medical Association included Doctors Daniel Meeker, Nathan Udell, John C. Jones, and Eugene B. Harrison. Other members of state societies were Doctors Meeker (Indiana, president), Anson Hurd (Indiana, Ohio), Udell (Iowa), Alexander M. Speer (Pennsylvania), Joseph S. Allen (Indiana), John C. Jones (Texas, vice president), Harrison (Ohio), and John E. L. Kimball (Maine). Doctors Samuel P. Moore and John C. Jones were members of the IX International Medical Congress. There is no corresponding list for the physician-generals.

A number of the control physicians were medical teachers. Doctor Albert Newman taught physiology at the University of Kansas for many years. Doctor David P. Smith was the Professor of the Theory and Practice of Medicine in Yale College from 1872 until his death in 1880. Doctor David McGugin was the Professor of Physiology, Pathology, and Microbiology at the College of Physicians and Surgeons, Keokuk and, for a time, also the president of the college. Doctor Daniel Meeker was a founder of the Indiana Medical College at LaPorte, the first medical school in the state. From 1842 to 1850, he taught variously anatomy, physiology, and surgery. This school graduated Doctor William W. Mayo, father of the Mayo brothers. Meeker later taught briefly at medical schools in Indianapolis and Keokuk. Doctor Duffee taught at an eclectic medical school in Philadelphia.

As judged by their return to the practice of medicine after the war, their interest in medical organizations, and their participation in teaching, the group of physician-generals had far less interest and success in medicine than did the control physicians.

Medical and Other Writing

The physician-generals wrote little on medicine but more on military subjects. This fact reflects their relative interests in these two fields. Besides the theses required by some schools for graduation and the medical and newspaper editing already mentioned, only Doctor Leasure contributed significantly to the medical and Elwell to the medico-legal literature. Myer's manual of signals was widely used *(Myer)*. To the war literature, Crawford's *Genesis of the Civil War* and Harris' book on the assassination of Lincoln were substantial historical contributions. Kimball and Leasure published papers on their military experiences, valuable because they are eyewitness accounts. Northrop wrote in the defense of his administration of the Confederate commissary department, and Blunt defended his military operations in Kansas and the adjoining areas *(Blunt)*. It is obvious that their war experiences had deeply impressed some of them. In addition, the wartime military writings of many of these officers, as published in the *Official Records,* are voluminous and historically valuable basic documents.

In addition to the usual quota of graduation theses, required at some of the better schools that had libraries, a number of the control physicians wrote official medical reports that were published in the *Official Records* or in the *Medical and Surgical History of the War of the Rebellion* (see Appendix of Part I, Volume I). In addition, Doctors D. P. Smith, McGugin, Meeker, Lyman, and Jones contributed a number of medical papers. Doctor Albert Newman published on the infectious diseases and on epidemiology. Perhaps George H. Lyman's writings were the most substantial from todays viewpoint. Beginning in 1854, when he won the Boylston prize in Boston for an essay on the nonmalignant diseases of the uterus, he wrote a series of papers, chiefly on gynecological conditions. Confederate Surgeon General Samuel P. Moore published a medical manual, and later was the president of the association of Confederate medical officers. After writing substantial medical papers, helping to found a medical school, and supporting medical organizations, Doctor Daniel Meeker wrote a tract, privately published in 1872, on opium eating, its consequences and cure *(Meeker)*. It passed through several editions. For this, he was expelled from the Indiana Medical Association for unethical conduct *(Russo),* five years before his death. The opium eating habit sometimes followed the prolonged treatment of chronic dysentery. Only in the writings of Doctors Newman and

Jones is there any evidence of their previous wartime medical experience.

Some members of Groups II and III also left substantial contributions, not only in the *Official Records,* but elsewhere. Of Group II, Generals Carr, Hartranft, and Page contributed eyewitness articles to the four-volume *Battles and Leaders of the Civil War.* General Michler published some professional engineering reports, and Lippitt lectured and wrote on military subjects as well as on his own adventurous life *(Lippitt).* General Logan, returning to national politics, wrote two books on war-related subjects. In one, he criticised the education at West Point *(Logan),* and in the other he tried to show the existence of a conspiracy by Southerners to destroy the Union (*Logan*). By today's standards, neither book is judicious. Leake contributed historical papers to volumes published by the Military Order of the Loyal Legion. General Walcott authored an interesting history of the Twenty-first Massachusetts Regiment *(Walcott).* Williams wrote for newspapers and magazines.

In Group III, Gorgas described the Confederate ordnance department *(Gorgas),* which he had so ably founded and developed. Doctors McDermont and Brown wrote medical reports of interest. General Brady, as an assistant postmaster-general, became involved in government mail scandals, and left a book to be published after his death—a legacy that has not been found.

In summary, the military and other writings of the physician-generals, while substantial, were not more impressive than those of the three control groups. Their medical writings were fewer than those of the control physicians. They were not exceptional officers by the criterion of authorship, and as physicians their published medical heritage is smaller than that of the controls.

Other Occupations

Among the physician-generals who returned to medicine after the war were a number who practiced briefly or part time. Not doing well from lack of interest or competence or because of poor health, they took other occupations. Doctors Cameron, Dustin, Harris, Miller, and Wentworth held various appointive sinecures and elective local, state, and federal positions. Blunt developed poor health and finally became a solicitor of claims in Washington. Cameron became a promoter in the west, Harris a part time farmer, Miller a bank cashier, and Capehart a part time druggist and coal dealer.

Among the nineteen who did not practice medicine were five who were partly disabled or semi-invalids—Lippincott, McMillen, Wainwright, Wild, Zulich—and one (Champion), who died soon. Two (Myer, Crawford) retained their military interests, and two (Brandon, Northrop) were in semi-retirement as planters, being the oldest men in the group. Three became carpet-baggers in the South: Catterson went to Arkansas, McMillen to Louisiana, and Scott to South Carolina. Although they were speculators or planters on the side, they did not prosper, even though Scott became a governor and McMillen an unseated senator. Gano became a clergyman and Harris sometimes preached. Most of the remainder were in law, politics, or business. Elwell and Leggett were prominent in the law.

The control physicians practically all returned to medicine. By this criterion, the two groups are strikingly different. The physician-generals, after the war, expanded their prewar record of multiple interests and diffusion of energies.

Longevity and Death

The thirty-three physician generals lived to an average age of sixty-nine years despite the early death of several from service-incurred diseases. The range was from thirty-two (Kiernan) to ninety-three (Harris) years. Doctor Bussey died in 1915, and nine others lived into the present century. Five died from causes related to their military service, and several others had disease conditions that might have been service-incurred. On the whole, however, life was not perceptibly shortened for this select group of survivors, the average life span having been like that of today. It is interesting that none had a diagnosis of neoplasm or of angina pectoris, although several had a history suggestive of the latter.

The average age of those members of the three control groups whose age at death is known was 65.9, 64.1, and seventy-one years. The ranges were, respectively, forty to eighty-eight, thirty-four to eighty-six, and forty-six to ninety-one years. The cause of death is not known for all, but in Group II no death was recognized as the sequel to a wartime disease. Several members of Group III died from war-related causes such as tuberculosis and dysentery. In Group IV, two died from tuberculosis (Hard, McGugin), at least two had persistent diarrhea (McGugin, Meeker), and one (Coolidge) had remittent fever. The death of several others was possibly service-related. Because of incomplete data and the small size of the four groups, it is not certain that the differences in survival time are statistically significant.

Chapter VII

SIGNIFICANCE OF PHYSICIANS IN COMBAT POSITIONS

SEVERAL FACTORS PROBABLY entered into the decision of each of these thirty-three physicians to serve in non-medical capacities. It is believed that the chief reason, already demonstrated to have been a factor, was:

(a) A weak commitment to medicine. This, in turn, was related to other factors including:
(b) The poor state of medical education.
(c) The underdeveloped condition of Medicine, both resulting in unattractiveness.
(d) The even greater unattractiveness of military medicine.
(e) Patriotism and belief in the cause.
(f) Leadership in community affairs.
(g) Ambition for military distinction.
(h) A spirit of restlessness and adventure.
(i) Miscellaneous reasons.

These factors may, on the whole, have been of decreasing importance in the order listed. Some of the influences existed or began in boyhood. They reflect, in part, the times in general but, to a greater degree, the special spirit and circumstances of that unusual war.

Weak Commitment to Medicine

It seems clear that an important factor in the decision of many of the thirty-three doctors was a *weak commitment to medicine.* Nine of them had abandoned medicine before the war, and nineteen did not practice after the war, while eight more practiced only part time, briefly, or intermittently. Some had gone from one occupation or profession to another, even several times. In all, they had tried forty-one other professions or occupations, not counting the military or those of their youth. They had shown little interest in the educational benefits of medical societies, in medical education, in publishing original medical observations, or in postdoctoral training for themselves. They had migrated and travelled extensively for nonmedical reasons.

All of these factors were different in the control physician group. Here, all had been in practice before the war and most of them returned to it afterward. They had not wandered from one profession to another or from place to place. Many of them supported medical organizations, some taught in medical schools, and a few had written on medical subjects.

Poor Medical Education

Some of these men seemed unsuited for or uninterested in medicine. Medical education prior to the war did not test for aptitude or sift out the unfitted, incompetent, or disinterested, and graduation did not require or confer a heavy commitment. A substantial premedical preparation was not required, and candidates were not screened. A few became physicians by serving only an apprenticeship, and others graduated after two short identical courses of lectures. Although the ability to practice well requires competence in acute observation and in recognition, the teaching was by lectures. Postdoctoral training was exceptional. Almost anybody could graduate, and proficiency was not tested or tested poorly prior to practice.

Education in a medical school was easily obtainable but it was not very good. Up to 1861, sixty-three recognized medical schools had been opened in the United States, and fifty of them were still in existence *(Billings)*. Forty of them were located in the Northern states, fourteen in what became the eleven states of the Confederacy, and nine were in the non-seceding four border slave states and the District of Columbia. Up to 1860, these schools had graduated 42,170 physicians, 35,890 of them in the three decades since 1830. To these must be added an unknown number who had only a apprenticeship. In as much as about 12,000 physicians served at one time or another in the medical department of the Union and 3,400 in the Confederate armies, it is apparent that a high proportion of the doctors of military age had army duty either in the medical departments or in the other capacities discussed in this volume. The doctors of the country were almost fully mobilized.

It is unlikely that the competent doctors entered the army and that the incompetent stayed at home, or that the reverse took place. It must be assumed that the physicians in the service in competence were representative of the profession as a whole.

Undeveloped and Unattractive State of Medicine

Medicine was *undeveloped and not very satisfying* in 1861 compared with later periods, which began explosively about 1880. Because of his poor education and the retarded state of medical knowledge, the graduate at best did not have much medical skill or power over disease. On graduation, he did not have a big investment in time, in skill, in energy, in money, or in emotions. Status and skill now came his way only to the degree that he won them by observation, intelligence, personality, industry, character, and ability. His economic condition might be poor, especially in rural communities where little money circulated and he had sometimes to accept payment in produce, where bank failures were common, and where he could see few patients in a day on horseback or by carriage. A new practice of sorts was not hard to come by so there was little restraint on migration or travel. A doctor had really to be dedicated to exert his full effort and interest. If he was unhappy, a change to another community, profession, or occupation was not difficult. The ease of making a change if things did not work out well might, in itself, have brought in some men without medical aptitude. The powers of the practitioner to prevent disease were almost nil; his ability to recognize and diagnose the diseases was somewhat better, but his curative powers were slight. His therapeutic efforts were mostly symptomatic and palliative, and Nature was his foremost therapeutic ally. Nearly all of his remedies have disappeared. His successes in practice were sure to be liberally larded with failures, so his satisfactions became diluted. The large number of young wives and children lost by these physicians themselves (see biographies) is eloquent evidence of the common powerlessness of medicine in the face of disease and disaster. One must admire the doctor who, without an anesthetic, could alone amputate a leg within minutes, but regret that simultaneously he unwittingly and inevitably contaminated the fresh stump he had just made—made sometimes for the purpose of removing infection.

It is difficult for us today to realize the medical conditions faced by the seventy-one physicians of this study. Of the infectious diseases, many could be diagnosed but only smallpox could be prevented, and this irregularly because of the variable potency and frequent secondary infection of the "vaccine matter," which could not be properly packaged. General Ben Butler made big political and military capital for himself by keeping yellow fever, which had made a frequent visitation, from New Orleans in the summer of 1862. Credit for this achievement properly belongs to his medical officer, Doctor Charles McCormick, who had adhered to the theory that the disease was not autogenous but that it came from without, and had, accordingly, enforced a strict quarantine on the river below the city. Historians have mistakenly attributed his success to cleaning out the open sewers and canals of the town and suppressing mosquitoes—both unnecessary and irrelevant if the virus was kept out. A major fatal infectious disease, tuberculosis, was not recognized as being transmissable, and a number of these doctors, as well as thousands of men, paid the penalty. No specific treatments were known. The nearest to that ideal was quinine for malaria. The degenerative, metabolic, cardiac, vascular, renal, nervous, muscular, skeletal, and other diseases had been only partly described, separated, and classified. Among the neoplasms, only the external types could be treated. The endocrine system and hormones were largely unknown. The only vitamin deficiency recognized was scurvy, but ideas on nutrition were primitive, so that even scurvy broke out a number of times in the army.

Diagnostic aids were few and clinical laboratories were unknown. The newest and most sophisticated diagnostic instrument of precision was the clinical thermometer; it was being tested for usefulness and was still in the "experimental stage." Many of the medical advances came from the morgue where the ultimate instruments of precision were the ruler and the balance, although free-hand sections made with a razor and examined unstained under the low power microscope were soon introduced. The hundreds of types of tests performed every day in our hospital laboratories, even simple blood counts, did not exist. One need only study a modern classification of disease to appreciate how many were unknown or incurable in those days. The leading causes of death of that day have almost disappeared from our mortality tables. Many physicians must have realized that their powers were weak and been unhappy at the fact.

Unattractive State of Military Medicine

Military medicine was even less attractive than medicine in general, and it is not surprising that so many physicians elected other types of service. Beside the undeveloped state of medicine in general was the special backwardness of military medicine, and the low status of the medical officer as an officer. The legal position of the doctor in uniform was poorly defined. In effect, the regimental surgeons were directly subordinate to the colonels. Moreover, their medical supply, personnel, and transportation services were often inadequate, and they had little control over their own medical facilities. The life was hard, and long periods of inactivity produced boredom and unhappiness. In the general hospitals of the rear areas, conditions were better, but few regimental surgeons were assigned to them. The medical officer, having little power over disease, wielded little military influence.

The medical aspects of the war have been presented from various viewpoints by many writers, both participants and reviewers *(Adams; Duncan; S.C. Gordon; A.G. Hall; Hart; Lyman, 1913)*. The special problems confronting Confederate medicine, resulting from its low potential in manufacturing drugs, books, and supplies, or in importing them consequent to the naval blockade, have also been described in detail *(Cunningham; Riley; Stark)*. These various points have been well documented and can be accepted here as established. Some aspects, pertinent to our present problem, require emphasis.

Medicine and the physicians were not very well prepared for the Civil War. The Mexican War had bequeathed no medical advances of importance, and none were made in the interim except for the introduction of anesthetics. One Indiana physician later wrote that of the five hundred surgeons enlisted from that state none in 1861 practiced surgery exclusively, most had never seen a major amputation, and few had treated gunshot wounds *(Kemper)*. Indianapolis, the capitol city, had no hospital. The situation in Indiana was not exceptional. The author emphasized the great psychological support the soldiers got from the great war songs. The boys needed support from those sad songs, but in World War II a corresponding support was not needed and the songs were not written. In the Confederate Army, also, nearly all of the surgeons had been general practitioners, unprepared for the vast problems of traumatic surgery *(Stark)*.

The legal status of the medical officer in the Civil War was not covered by legislation *(Woodhull)*. His duties might be great but his authority was not. In training camp, in the field, or in battle his best efforts might be heroic but they were not very effective. During recruitment, his ability soundly to accept or disqualify was limited. Despite the regulations he often took these examinations lightly. In camp, when the infectious diseases invariably and promptly broke out, he could do little. If the several million cases of diarrhea and dysentery were preventable at that time, their occurrence would be a terrible indictment of the military surgeons. He successfully treated intermittent swamp fever with quinine, but unfortunately wasted some of this precious drug on other fevers. We regard tincture of opium a poor substitute for sulfa drugs in acute enteritis, but it was the best he had. Field sanitation and personal hygiene were primitive. The importance of sewage, garbage, animal offal, manure, and dead horse and mule disposal, of insect and rodent control, of food and water protection and purification were largely unknown. The Battle of Perryville, with its 7,607 casualties in a few hours, developed one afternoon over competition among thirsty soldiers in a drought area for the precious remaining green-scummed water holes in a drying Kentucky creek. The Lyster bag came much later, after chemical sterilization was known.

The surgeon was variously welcomed, accepted, or tolerated. He might become a close personal friend of the commander, but he was not a very important member of his staff. He could not serve on courts-martial *(Woodhull)*. Experienced campaigners knew that their command was healthier if kept moving and that camps should be policed. They could also calculate the anticipated percentage attrition in their command by disease according to season, location, and length of prior service of their troops without help from their medical officer. Sherman, whose actions and evolution of ideas can be traced almost day by day because of the enormous volume of correspondence he left, and who must be credited for much originality in thinking, owed little to his medical officers. His working classification of disease, expressed already in 1863 to Grant, was simple *(O.R. 138):* "We have a good deal of real sickness and still more of that sort which develops on the approach of danger." Actually, his working classification was far more sophisticated than that. He knew that man could live for a time on meat and salt alone, so he was less afraid than others of being cut off from his base, knowing that if necessary they could subsist on their mules and artillery, cavalry, ambulance, and private horses.

The regimental surgeon was handicapped from the day he enlisted under the colonel. He was selected or approved by the colonel, and commissioned by the governor for duty in a specified regiment. He could resign and re-enlist, but not transfer if conditions were bad. He took his orders from the colonel or brigadier, and had practically no contacts with the medical department in Washington. The commanders might be ignorant both militarily and medically, but they wielded the day-to-day power. Brigadier Hanson, a young lawyer, suspecting that the men of his brigade were malingering, issued an order that there should be only two sick men at one time in each company *(Duke)!*

The surgeon's troubles often began with the pre-mustering physical examinations. Three men—the colonel, the U. S. mustering officer, and the surgeon, if appointed—conducted this examination with various degree of dominance and skill. At some, the surgeon had no influence. This muster may have been preceded by an enlistment examination, for which some men were not even requested to undress. The state medical departments had made little or no provision for the measles, mumps, and diarrheas that usually began in the camps of assembly, often a county fair-ground. Over the sanitary and hygienic arrangements and the diet for the regiment during its transportation and in camp, the surgeon often had little control. His effectiveness in enforcing the regulations on camp sanitation depended directly on his support by the colonel *(Curtis)*. He was expected by many commanders to be present on the battlefield, where he was essentially a corpsman. Sometimes, however, he acted as an aide to the colonel in carrying orders. Dozens of commendations published in the official post-action reports testify to this duty. Medical corpsmen did not exist as trained aides on the field or as nurses in the hospital. The medical supply situation in campaigns was often as bad as that of the general supplies, and sometimes worse (*Gordon; Gunn*). Before Gettysburg, General Meade ordered all wagon trains except ammunition and medical kept well to the rear of the army, but the quartermaster held back the medical wagons, except in the Twelfth Corps. In three days the Union doctors were confronted by 14,529 wounded, and 3,155 more mortally wounded; the Confederates, some of whom came under the care of the Union surgeons, were about the same. The result was not pleasant. Just before Shiloh Grant pleaded for important medicines for 10,000 sick, some of them weeks overdue *(O.R. 10: (2) 57, 73)*.

Doctor Moses Gunn, then of Ann Arbor but later in Chicago, expressed the feelings of many surgeons when he wrote to his wife in 1862 from the Army of the Potomac, after complaining of his inability to get supplies and equipment *(Gunn)*:

> "I have been marching and counter-marching, in heat, in cold, in wet, in hunger, in anger, in ignorance and despair, at the beck and nod of others, until the thing is about 'played out.' I have never felt so small, so insignificant, in short so *mean,* as I have since I have been a *thing* to be ordered about."

Soon, on July 1st, he became bedridden in his ambulance (i.e., wagon). He had been without adequate food for some days when he was found on the 11th by his twelve-year-old son. The boy went to where beef was being killed but the supply was exhausted. He finally found some liver adherent to discarded entrails which he cut off with his pocket knife and carried to his bedridden father, who soon resigned.

When the colonel of the Forty-fourth Indiana at Pittsburg Landing complained that too many men fit for duty were being excused, the surgeon suggested that the colonel and the chaplain, who had formerly been a physician, themselves hold sick call. They found hardly a man in the regiment free from diarrhea and other diseases, and the criticism stopped *(Rerich)*. Such an effective solution to criticism was rarely possible. But the fact remains that there was much disease, which the doctor was powerless to control.

In fact, the rare regiments that failed to develop the expected high incidence of camp diseases attracted unwelcome attention and trouble for the surgeons. The Thirteenth Iowa was twice inspected under a suspicion of falsification of its medical reports (*Thrall*). Over a period of two years it had an unprecedented low morbidity and mortality in the generally unhealthy Second Corinth, Western Tennessee, Vicksburg, and Meridian Campaigns. Its prevalence rates of camp diseases were about one-fourth those of the other three regiments in Crocker's Iowa Brigade, in the division, and in the Army of the Tennessee. In one period of nine months of living in swamps and on the Mississippi levee, there were only four deaths. Inspections were made first by the divisional medical director and, some months later, by a medical inspector sent from Washington. Assistant Surgeon Thrall attributed the low rates to a more judicious use of quinine and whiskey and to the avoidance of calomel and drastic cathartics. These measures might explain a low mortality but they could not have accounted for the low rate of infection, and the mystery remains.

Consequently, except for the big surgical experience after the occasional battles, there were few rewards for the medical officers apart from the gratitude of the boys for faithful service. The uncontrollable epidemics, poor medical facilities, and abundant paper work were unattractive. The constant presence of silent cases or chronic carriers of typhoid fever, dysentery, malaria, tuberculosis, meningitis, streptococcic infections, and others, gave rise to epidemics regardless of the type of camp policing. Flies, lice, mosquitoes, and other disease vectors, overcrowding in the hovels used in the winter camps, and the contaminated water supplies tended to negate the effectiveness of the sanitary measures taken. Bacteriological cleanness was an unformulated concept and gross cleanness by itself was not effective. The drinking water from a clear cool stream might, unknown to them, be a dangerous bacterial culture, while the water from a dirty pond containing dead mules might be safe. On the march it was standard procedure to order a ten minute rest every hour. Diarrheic bowels required frequent relief more than muscles needed rest, and they had to be relieved even if the men had to straggle to do so. It was soon found that many men did not have the "guts" for soldiering, but in this matter a physician was no better informed and little more effective than anybody else, as is evidenced by the diseases in the seventy-one physicians of this study. One colonel went so far as to call the fecal odor that developed around every camp a "patriotic odor" as it would persist as long as a patriot remained in the army *(J. R. Bowen)*.

In neither medical department were the administrative and organizational measures taken promptly to meet the needs of the large scale warfare that developed. The Federal army, increasing from 16,000 to over 1,000,000 within a year, brought together great numbers of disease susceptibles. There was no equivalent expansion in the army hospital or medical plant. Consequently, there were times when the application of the existing medical knowledge, inadequate even as it was, was not fully used. In the Peninsular Campaign of 1862, at Shiloh, at Second Bull Run, and elsewhere, the medical care fell short of needs and knowledge. Surgeons Hammond, Letterman and many others were unhappy with the situation and a few heads rolled. The failure to control disease even late in the war is shown by an official report. On March 1, 1865, the Union Army numbered 965,591 men, of whom 602,598 were present for duty and 362,993 absent or sick *(O.R. 140)*. The latter figure included 143,449 men absent in general hospitals or sick at home, and 35,628 sick in field hospitals or unfit for duty. Tens of thousands more were dead, had received medical discharges, had simply gone home, or were sick in camp. After four years of experience on a vast scale with the control of diseases, great numbers were dead or had been discharged as disabled, yet over one-third of those on the rolls were ineffective. New regiments raised in 1864 shrank away from disease about as fast as those enrolled in 1861.

Although some of the unattractiveness of military medicine came from the very nature of army life and operations in that day, a sizable part came from the inadequacy of medical supplies, equipment, plant, and personnel. Nobody in charge foresaw, or perhaps could have foreseen, the enormous medical expansion that would be needed to service the unpredictably large armies. This blindness was not limited to the army medical department. The transactions of the annual meetings of the American Medical Association through 1860 give no hint that the nation was on the verge of a great war

(*Fishbein*). After the inadequacies had developed, however, the medical profession supported expansion in military medical personnel and supplies, authority adequate to meet the problems, and the elimination of incompetent doctors. The medical periodicals of that day published many informative and critical communications of current interest. The voluntary Sanitary Commission provided relief to the soldiers on a large scale and it exerted great pressure on the War Department for good.

One complaint of the surgeons about military surgery was that they could not learn much scientifically from their work. They could gain skill of hand in operations but not in surgical judgment because the end results were lost to them. After large battles, the patients were evacuated from the field and boat hospitals, where most of the surgery was performed, to the rear general hospitals, where they came into other hands. Surgeon Edmund Andrews, Professor of Surgery in Lind University, Chicago, complained that the scientific results from the battles of Fort Donelson, Shiloh, and Corinth had thus been lost *(Andrews, 1863)*. By strenuous efforts and initiative, he was able to set up a system whereby the fate of the wounds in the battle at Chickasaw Bluffs could be observed and recorded for a period of at least twenty days. This seems to have been the first systematic surgical research of its type during the war.

It is unlikely, however, that dissatisfaction with the army medical corps played a predominant part in the decisions of the doctors here studied because most of them had made their decision before some of the deficiencies had appeared. However, the general unattractiveness of army medicine must have been widely known.

Patriotism and Belief in the Cause

Most of these physician-generals enlisted soon after the attack on Fort Sumter, a time when patriotism flared to a peak on both sides. In the North, the shelling was followed by ringing bells, closed schools and businesses, and patriotic meetings in nearly every community. In the South, feeling had already been running high for some weeks in the seven seceded cotton states, and it quickly rose in four states of the Upper South when the call was made on them for troops to put down the rebellion. As after the attack on Pearl Harbor in 1941, the issues were quickly simplified, clarified, and accepted. In the North, it became a matter of the attack on the flag and restoration of the Union; the slavery issues temporarily faded into the background. To the Southerners, the issue clearly, for the time, became one of defending their constitutional rights and liberties and repelling an invader.

Most of the early enlistments took place under these conditions. Because the affair would end quickly, physicians could enlist as combat soldiers as little surgery would be needed. The political issues had been before the country since 1820, and intensively and almost constantly discussed since 1850. Every citizen was familiar with them. They had repeatedly been election issues (unlike the situation in 1941) in one form or another since the Birney abolition ticket in 1840.

Powerful psychological factors played an important part in that war. On both sides, it was fought with great doggedness. The hardships withstood during active operations and in winter camps were, at times, unbelievable. Many men remained in service with a wound or disease that today would be a ticket home or out. When General Hancock, himself a victim of serious war-incurred osteomyelitis, left the Second Corps at Petersburg in the autumn of 1864 to raise a new Invalid Corps of veterans, he found many ready to reenlist for limited service. Nobody knows how many of the men marching up Pennsylvania Avenue in the Victory Parade had chronic amebic or bacillary dysentery but it may have been a majority in some units. The men on both sides were familiar with the issues, and they were deeply committed. The strength they derived from their convictions was a priceless military asset in adversity. The respect they gained from each other made it possible for them to share the food in their haversacks at Appomattox. These doctors must have shared in this general feeling.

The political views of the thirty-three who became generals have already been mentioned insofar as they are known. Some of the twenty-seven who became Federal generals were strong Unionists, others abolitionists, and still others were both. Undoubtedly the six Southerners reflected the interests and beliefs of their section.

Patriotism and belief in the cause must have swayed some of these doctors to enlist, and a misunderstanding of the magnitude and duration the war would assume probably caused some of them to volunteer as infantry and cavalrymen rather than as surgeons. The service with Negro troops, for which a few of them later volunteered, suggests sympathy for the suppressed on the part of some, as does their staying on after the war in the Freedman's Bureau. In other instances, these decisions may have been made on the basis of personal ambition.

That war was like a crusade in which everybody knew that the issues were important even if he did not understand all of their ramifications. A bit of the old chivalry still existed at the beginning, but it rapidly disappeared under the hard warfare that evolved. On both sides, most of the participants were volunteers. As the bitter struggle continued, resistance and determination hardened. Few liked soldiering but the ultimate objectives kept them going. In 1864, a higher proportion of Union soldiers voted for the reelection of Lincoln than in some of the corresponding civilian populations, although they understood that his reelection meant more fighting and dying, which would fall to their lot. These doctors contributed their patriotic ardor to the general pool.

Leadership in Community Affairs

Most of the troops were recruited by companies or regiments in the communities under state authorization. A leading citizen, who was either self-appointed or designated by higher authority, could open and conduct the enlistment. As is seen in the biographies in Chapter III, this local leader was sometimes the doctor. As an educated, responsible, and travelled man, the physician was among the community elders. Moreover, many of the future physician-generals were especially well fitted for community leadership because they had been in politics, had legal, business or other experience, or had a little military training. It was natural for the boys to elect the doctor and for him to accept even if he had originally intended to serve as a surgeon. The country, in 1861, had few men with military education to officer the regiments, so the officers would have to learn their profession while on the job. An intelligent physician could do this as well as other men.

Personal Ambition for Military Distinction

Personal ambition and a desire for military distinction may have influenced some of these doctors to become non-medical officers. This motive was attributed to Crawford by one of his Fort Sumter brother officers, and to Capehart. As regimental medical officers with volunteers, these thirty-three doctors could not go far. Their military status was below that of the lowest officer of field grade—the major of the regiment. They could aspire to the grade of brigade surgeon, but this also carried only the equivalent rank of major. In contrast, in positions of combat leadership, their aspirations need have no limit. Usually, men would not admit this motive, and its importance can only be guessed. It is my belief that several of the thirty-three were influenced by this factor but that it was relatively unimportant. The postwar life of many of the thirty-three discloses ambition other than medical, but neither was it then military.

If extrapolation to these physician-generals is permitted from the experience of some other physicians who chose non-medical positions, additional evidence can be brought to bear. For example, Doctor Edward W. Cade, aged twenty-three, a graduate at Jefferson in 1858, declined an offer as assistant surgeon in Richmond and was elected a lieutenant in a Texas cavalry regiment. After serving for nearly six months, during which time he had several attacks of diarrhea, he went before a second army medical board. Offered a commission as surgeon with the rank of major, he now accepted *(Anderson, 1957)*.

The biographies in Chapter III characterize the military service performed by these physician-generals. The medical histories of these officers and of the members of the other three groups in camp and battle characterize the state of military medicine practiced at the time. From them can be judged which profession would give the greater satisfaction to the participant. The conclusion arrived at would depend on the objectives in life of the individual. To some this may have been military glory more than medical satisfaction.

For making a decision on the relative attractiveness of the combat versus the medical positions, the final hard outcome should be recognized lest these doctors be judged too harshly:

(a) Among the hundreds of physicians who began their service in the infantry and later transferred to the medical department, *none* reached general rank.

(b) Among the approximately fifteen thousand volunteer physicians in medical departments, *one* reached general grade by brevet, after the war.

(c) Among the few dozens of physicians who began their service in the medical department and later transferred to a combat position, *five* reached general rank.

(d) Among the few thousand physicians who began their service in the infantry, cavalry, etc. and remained in the non-medical services, *twenty-eight* reached general rank.

These facts were not known to the thirty-three physicians of Group I when they made their decision, but the underlying conditions that determined this outcome were observable to a keen analyst and observer.

The military correspondence left by many of these physician-generals was small in amount considering their rank. This fact shows that they were not glory-seekers or militarily ambitious. One way to win recognition from above was to submit favorable post-action reports whenever possible. The same report could later be leaked back to the newspaper in the writer's community, where it would bring local military fame. Military correspondence, substituting for oral communication, could be used in the same ways. Many of the physician-generals did not use these devices. For example, Doctor Capehart went from surgeon to brevet major general at Appomattox without leaving a single official report. Others have a similar record. This is not the behavior of self-seekers.

Spirit of Adventure

Most of the physician-generals enlisted in April and May of 1861 when it looked as if the war would be short. The first Union call for troops was for only ninety days. Many thought there would be one battle at most. Under these conditions, the *spirit of adventure* might well have been a factor in enlistment. By their migration westward,

TABLE V

SOME REPRESENTATIVE PHYSICIANS AS FIELD GRADE OFFICERS—UNION

Name	*Regiment***	*Comments*	*References*
Lieutenant Colonel John C. Abercrombie	Eleventh Iowa	Wounded at Shiloh	Byers; Ware
Colonel Moses M. Bane	Fiftieth Illinois	Lost arm at Shiloh	Wilson
Colonel James M. Brown	One Hundredth New York	Killed at Fair Oaks	Stowits
Major James H. Carpenter	Seventh Indiana Cavalry	Also a lawyer	Cogley
Colonel Theodore Spencer Case	Quartermaster-Gen. of Mo.		C.A.B.
Brevet Colonel Charles W. Clancy	Fifty-second Ohio		Stewart
Colonel William W. Dewey	Twenty-third Iowa	Died of erysipelas, 1862	Stuart
Colonel Norman Eddy	Forty-eighth Indiana		Indiana Soldiers
Colonel Charles R. Ellet	Comdr. "Queen of the West"	Died of a "swamp disease"	Bates
Brevet Colonel Moses S. Hall	Tenth West Virginia		Matheny
Colonel George S. Hays	Thirty-seventh Pennsylvania	Resigned for ill health, 1862	Bates
Major S. M. Hewett	Thirty-second Ohio		O.R. 141
Colonel Asher S. Leidy	Ninety-ninth Pennsylvania	Wounded at Fredericksburg	Bates
Colonel James M. Lewis	Twenty-eighth Wisconsin		J. M. Lewis
Colonel John W. Lyman	Two Hundred and Third Pa.	Killed in assault at Fort Fisher	Martin *et al.*
Lieutenant Colonel Samuel Marsh	Sixteenth New York	Died of Wounds, 1862	Curtis
Colonel Francis Moro	Sixty-third Illinois	Also a clergyman	Wilson
Colonel John W. Moss	Fifth West Virginia Cavalry	Resigned in 1862	Reader
Major Louis H. Naghel	Eighty-third Pennsylvania	Killed by shrapnel, Gaines' Mill	Bates
Lieutenant Colonel Solomon A. Paddock	Ninth Illinois Cavalry	Died suddenly in 1862	Davenport
Major Bowman H. Peterson	Twenty-ninth Missouri	Disabled at Crump's Landing	Powell
Colonel Hugh B. Reed	Forty-fourth Indiana	Resigned for ill health, 1862	Rerich
Colonel William W. Ricketts	Sixth Pennsylvania Reserves	Died of Lung Hemorrhage, 1862	Sypher
Major Robert G. Rider	Eighty-fifth Illinois	Gunshot wound in head, 1864	Aten
Colonel George Ryan	Seventy-fifth Illinois	Helped surgeon while under arrest	Eddy
Lieutenant Colonel Lucius M. Sargent, Jr.	First Massachusetts Cavalry	Killed in 1864	Gleason
Colonel Joseph Thoburn	First West Virginia	Wounded, 1862; killed, 1864	Rawling
Lieutenant Colonel James P. Walker	Eighty-fifth Illinois	Formerly regimental surgeon	Aten
Colonel John Ward	Twelfth New York		Dowley
Colonel William C. Williams	Forty-fourth Indiana	Resigned, 1863	Rerick

*All were U. S. Volunteers.

**Regiments were infantry unless otherwise specified.

TABLE VI

SOME REPRESENTATIVE PHYSICIANS AS FIELD OFFICERS—CONFEDERATE

Name	*Regiment**	*Comments*	*References*
Major James F. Beall	Twenty-first North Carolina	Wounded five times	Beall
Lieutenant Colonel Elbert Bland	Seventh South Carolina	Killed at Chickamauga	Dickert
Colonel J. B. Davis	Fifteenth South Carolina		Dickert
Colonel W. L. Duckworth	Seventh Tennessee Cavalry	Served under Forrest	Henry
Lieutenant Colonel Thomas C. Glover	Twenty-first Georgia	Killed at Winchester, 1864	Thomas
Lieutenant Colonel F. S. Lewis	Fifteenth South Carolina		Dickert
Lieutenant Colonel R. W. Martin	Fifty-third Virginia	Wounded and captured at Gettysburg	Martin
Lieutenant Colonel James M. McLaughlin	Eighteenth Alabama		McLaughlin
Colonel Thomas M. Nelson	Mississippi regiment	Killed in 1865	Thomas
Colonel J. W. Starnes	Fourth Tennessee Cavalry	Killed in 1863	Wyeth

*Infantry regiments unless otherwise specified.

practice in frontier communities, travel to the isolated and new west coast, and service in Mexico and the Crimea, a number of these doctors had previously given way to a spirit of adventure. Now, because there would be little or no fighting, medical officers would find little to do and doctors had best quickly join up in any capacity.

Although the spirit of adventure might initially have been a factor for some, it was ultimately not important because they remained in service, unless incapaciteted by poor health, long after adventure had fled and soldiering became tough. As officers, they could have resigned, but only a few did.

Miscellaneous Factors

Suggestions have been made that some enlisted to escape *difficult domestic situations,* nagging wives, and family responsibilities. No evidence has been found in these officers for this factor. A safe, quiet refuge could have been found more easily in a medical than in a non-medical assignment. Neither is there any evidence that these doctors avoided or failed to gain medical commissions because of *medical incompetence.* None of them had failed before a medical examining board, state or federal, as far as is known. The five who began their military service as physicians and transferred later seem to have been medically competent while they served.

Additional Physicians as Officers of Field Grade

The phenomenon of physicians serving in non-medical capacities is further shown to have been common by the lists of thirty Union officers of field grade in Table V and of ten Confederates of these ranks in Table VI. These tables were compiled with little effort. They include only a small proportion of the physicians acting in the capacities of colonel, lieutenant colonel, and major. Some of these officers came to my attention because of their wounds and illnesses. No doubt these disabilities prevented some of them from becoming general officers.

Chapter VIII

GENERALS FROM THE OTHER PROFESSIONS

MEDICINE WAS NOT exceptional in contributing combat officers. All of the professions—law, education, engineering, theology, dentistry, and others—provided line and field grade officers in addition to filling the few available army positions peculiar to the specialty. Lawyers were in great surplus and hundreds became officers in the infantry, cavalry, and artillery. Many of them had also been politicians, and they were leaders in the communities. Teachers of all kinds, from grade school to universities, enlisted in great numbers. In the South, especially, the faculties of the colleges became badly depleted and some schools were closed. Many engineers became army engineers but others had duty in the infantry or cavalry, dividing, in this respect, like the physicians and the officers in the regular army corps of engineers. One dentist, Byron Root Pierce, was commissioned a brigadier general in 1864 and a brevet major general later. He had been wounded five times and had lost a leg. As a specialty, dentistry was then in its infancy.

Among clergymen, the situation gradually evolved much as it did for physicians. Many enlisted as chaplains and others as privates and officers. Some members of both groups crossed over. A number became general officers. Three well known examples in the Confederate service were Lieutenant General Leonidas Polk, Brigadier General Mark P. Lowrey, and Brigadier General William N. Pendleton. All three continued to perform occasional ministerial duties. Polk, a friend of Davis' and an Episcopal bishop, led a corps up to the time of his death under Sherman's guns at Pine Mountain, Georgia in June, 1864. Pendleton, the chief of artillery of the Army of Northern Virginia, was said to have named the four guns of his first battery Matthew, Mark, Luke, and John. At Appomattox he was one of the three Confederate officers designated by Lee to carry out the stipulations of the terms of surrender. Polk and Pendleton were old West Point graduates from 1827 and 1830. Bishop Polk likened his military role to that of a clergyman helping, in the emergency, firemen extinguish a great fire.

In the Federal army, the Reverend William A. Pile, a Methodist minister, became a chaplain early in 1861, a captain of artillery in 1862, a colonel later that year, and a brigadier general in 1863. After the war, he was brevetted a major general *(Warner)*. Many ministers won brevets to brigadier general. These include former Chaplain James C. Beecher of New York *(C.A.B.)*, Hasbrouck Davis of the Twelfth Illinois Cavalry, and Chaplain John Eaton *(C.A.B.)*, who served Grant so ably as the superintendent of freedmen in the Mississippi valley. Chaplain Samuel Fallows was with various Wisconsin units before he became the colonel of the Forty-ninth Regiment and, later, a brigadier *(B.D.A.)*. Colonel Granville Moody (and Reverend) was discharged for disability from four wounds received at the battle of Stone's River and awarded the higher grade *(C.A.B.)*. The Reverend Jesse Hale Moore led a brigade in the Army of the Cumberland *(C.A.B.)*. Chaplain Eliphalet Whittlesey won various staff positions in the Nineteenth Maine and finally the colonelcy of the Forty-sixth U. S. Colored Infantry and a brevet brigadiership *(Heitman)*. Most of these eight general officers had a college education and some had taken special theological courses as well. None had previous military training. Some of them had also been in the field of education. Four of the eight (Pile, Beecher, Eaton, Whittelsey) led colored troops during the war. With respect to this choice of duty, they were like the physician group.

At lower ranks, the number of clergymen who became colonels of national infantry regiments is large. An incomplete list includes Colonels Eber C. Byam of the Twenty-fourth Iowa, John B. Clark of the One Hundred and Twenty-third Pennsylvania, Jeremiah C. Drake of the One Hundred and Twelfth New York, William Batchelder of the First Massachusetts Heavy Artillery, James J. Jaquess of the Seventy-third Illinois, James M. McCarter of the Ninety-third Pennsylvania, David Hastings Moore of the One Hundred and Twenty-fifth Ohio, James H. Perry of the Forty-eighth New York, and James Pike of the Sixteenth New Hampshire. Some of these ministers would have received higher grade had their career not been interrupted by wounds or disease. Thus, Colonel Byam resigned in 1863 for illness, Drake was killed in action at Cold Harbor in 1864, McCarter was wounded at Fair Oaks in 1862, and Perry died of apoplexy in 1862.

The enthusiasm and support of the clergy were such that entire regiments with a large quota of ministers were enlisted in some states. The Seventy-third Illinois was known as the "Preacher" or "Methodist" Regiment. It was largely recruited in the dark days of July, 1862 by preachers, and the overflow was so great that preachers from this regiment helped to form the One Hundred and Fifteenth and the One Hundred and Seventeenth Illinois *(Historical Committee)*. The One Hundred and Twenty-fourth Illinois was known as the "Temperance" regiment. It contained eleven ordained and five licensed ministers; five of them were commissioned officers besides the chaplain *(Howard)*. In the Twenty-fourth Iowa, also known as the "Methodist" or "Temperance" regiment, the colonel and a number of the captains were ministers *(Ely)*.

Among the 583 Union general officers of full rank who served during the war, 126 were lawyers or jurists, twenty-six were civil engineers, and sixteen were educators *(Warner)*. The corresponding figures for 425 Confederate generals were 129 lawyers and jurists, fifteen educators, thirteen civil engineers, and three ministers. The numbers of professional soldiers, in contrast, were 194 Federal and 125 Confederates. Business men, farmers, politicians, doctors, and students accounted for most of the remainder. The war was well supported by the professional men of all kinds, and many of them moved into the combat officer class when military leadership was needed on a large scale.

Chapter IX

MULTIPLE PROFESSIONS

JUST AS MANY OF THE physician-generals had tried a number of different vocations, so had many of the officers coming from the other professions. A change from one profession to another was a common phenomenon in that period of our history. The men of all professions in 1860, like the doctors, had only a small educational investment in time, finances, and energy. The educational prerequisites for admission to professional schools was low, and most professions could also be entered without attendance at a recognized school. Almost anybody could become a politician. By reading law in an office for a few months, one had a new profession. The educational requirements for teachers and the clergy, like those for physicians, were often minimal. Many of the best engineers came from West Point, but here engineering subjects comprised only a small part of the curriculum, and the admission requirements were low by the standards of today.

It was easy to go from one profession to another until one found his niche, so many people tried two or more. President William Henry Harrison thus abandoned medicine for the military life and, finally, politics. Even Doctor Benjamin Rush, after ten years of practice, had planned to take up law when the evacuation of Philadelphia by the British army caused him to return to his old practice *(Corner)*. Many of the West Point graduates who became prominent during the war had resigned from the army and taken up other professions. The examples of Bishop Polk, Reverend Pendleton, Doctor Northrop and others have already been mentioned. Sherman had graduated in 1840 and resigned in 1853 as a commissary in the grade of captain. Thereafter he was a banker in San Francisco and New York (1853-1857), a lawyer in Leavenworth, Kansas (1858-1859), the superintendent of the state military academy of Louisiana (1859-1861), and the president of a horse-car railroad in St. Louis (1861) before re-entering the army as the colonel of the new Thirteenth U. S. Infantry *(Sherman)*.

A few other examples of combinations of professions in men who were in the war were Colonel W. L. Duckworth of Forrest's cavalry who had been both a preacher and physician (*Henry*) and Colonel Francis Moro of the Sixty-third Illinois who had the same professions. Colonel John Borland of the One Hundred and Third Pennsylvania was both a clergyman and lawyer. Brevet Brigadier General Walter Harriman of New Hampshire had been a teacher, minister, politician, and editor before he became a soldier. James F. Jacquess was a lawyer, preacher, teacher, and chaplain before he was elected the colonel of the Seventy-third Illinois. He had also been the president of the Illinois Female College and of Quincy College. Colonel James H. Perry had practiced law in New York, been a cadet at West Point for three years, fought in the Texas war for independence, and had finally become a Methodist clergyman. His second military career was ended by death in June, 1864 at Fort Pulaski, Georgia. Brevet Major General Green Clay Smith of Kentucky, a nephew of politician and General Cassius M. Clay, was a private soldier in Mexico, a lawyer and a politician before he became a private in 1861 and a brigadier in 1862. After the war he was again a politician and, finally, a Baptist minister. Brevet Brigadier General Hasbrouck Davis had been a teacher, minister, and lawyer. Colonel William Bachelder had been a non-graduating cadet at West Point, a lieutenant in the Seminole War, and a clergyman.

Many other examples of the easy and frequent shift from one profession to another could be cited. The situation at that stage of our history was quite unlike the rigidity and frozen conformity in the professions today. To such men who had already professed if not mastered several occupations, the adoption of still another one during the country's dire trial was not a big jump. It is clear that medicine was not unique in failing to retain all of its professors.

ORIGINS OF THE ILLUSTRATIONS

1. Anderson—Miller, F.T., Editor: *Photographic History of the Civil War.* Vol. 10. New York, Review of Reviews, 1911, p. 261.
2. Blunt—*Ibid.:* p. 175.
3. Brandon—*Ibid.:* p. 277.
4. Bratton—La Bree, Ben, Editor: *Confederate Soldier in the Civil War.* Louisville, Prentice Press, 1897, p. 371.
5. Brown—Library of Congress.
6. Bussey—Powell, W.H.: *Officers of the Army and Navy (Volunteer) Who Served in the Civil War.* Philadelphia, Hamersly, 1893.
7. Cameron—Library of Congress.
8. Capehart—Lang, T.F.: *Loyal West Virginia from 1861 to 1865.* Baltimore, Deutsch, 1895, p. 164.
9. Catterson—Miller, F.T.: *op. cit.,* p. 203.
10. Champion—Partridge, C.A., Editor: *History of the Ninety-Sixth Regiment Illinois Volunteer Infantry.* Chicago, Historical Society of the Regiment, 1887.
11. Crawford—Bates, S.P.: *Martial Deeds of Pennsylvania.* Philadelphia, Davis, 1876, p. 810.
12. Dustin—Hard, A.: *History of the Eighth Cavalry Regiment Illinois Volunteers.* Aurora (no publisher), 1868, p. 239.
13. Elliott—*Companions of the Military Order of the Loyal Legion of the U.S.* New York, Hamersly, 1901.
14. Elwell—Library of Congress.
15. Gano—Miller, F.T.: *op. cit.,* p. 315.
16. Harris—Lang, T.F.: *op. cit.,* p. 323.
17. Hillis—Library of Congress.
18. Kiernan—Library of Congress.
19. Kimball—Partridge, C.A.: *op. cit.,* p. 240.
20. Leasure—Bates, S.P.: *op. cit.,* p. 628.
21. Leggett—Reid, W.: *Ohio in the War.* Vol. 1. Cincinnati, Moore, Wilstack, and Baldwin, 1868, p. 617.
22. Lippincott—Elliott, I.H., and Way, V.G.: *History of the Thirty-Third Regiment Illinois Veteran Volunteer Infantry.* Gibson City, Published by the Association, 1902, p. 8.
23. Ludlow—Reid, W.: *op. cit.,* p. 951.
24. McMillen—Library of Congress.

25. Miller—Magee, B.F.: *History of the Seventy-Second Indiana Volunteer Infantry.* Lafayette, Vater, 1882, Frontispiece.
26. Myer—Brown, J.W.: *The Signal Corps, U.S.A., in the War of the Rebellion.* Boston, U.S. Veteran Signal Corps Association, 1896, Frontispiece.
27. Northrop—Warner, E.J.: *Generals in Gray.* Baton Rouge, Louisiana State University Press, 1959, p. 225.
28. Robertson—Miller, F.T.: *loc. cit.*
29. Scott—Miller, F.T.: *op. cit.,* p. 237.
30. Wainwright—Smith, A.P.: *History of the Seventy-Sixth Regiment New York Volunteers.* Cortland, Printed for the Publisher, 1867, p. 348.
31. Wentworth—Houston, H.C.: *The Thirty-Second Maine Regiment of Infantry Volunteers.* Portland, Southworth, 1903, p. 48.
32. Wild—Bowen, J.L.: *Massachusetts in the War.* Springfield, Bryan, 1889, p. 1009.
33. Zulich—Bates, S.P.: *op. cit.,* p. 468.

BIBLIOGRAPHY

A. General References

Adjutant General's Reports, 1861-1866, of the concerned state.

Army Registers, Official, of the Regular and Volunteer Forces. Washington, Adjutant General's Office, 1860-1865.

Atkinson, W. B.: *The Physicians and Surgeons of the United States.* Philadelphia, Robson, 1878, 788 pp.

Biographical Dictionary of America. Edited by R. Johnson, and J. H. Brown. Boston, Amer. Biographical Society, 10 vols., 1906 (abbr. as "BDA").

Cullum, G. W.: *Biographical Register of the Officers and Graduates of the U. S. Military Academy at West Point,* 3rd Ed. New York, Van Nostrand, 3 vols., 1891.

Cyclopaedia of American Biography. Edited by J. G. Wilson, and J. Fiske. New York, Appleton, 6 vols., 1887 (abbr. as "CAB").

Dictionary of American Biography. Edited by A. Johnson. New York, Scribner, 20 vols., 1928-1937 (abbr. as "DAB").

Evans, C. A., Editor: *Confederate Military History.* Atlanta, Confederate, 12 vols., 1899.

Fox, W. F.: *Regimental Losses in the American Civil War, 1861-1865.* Albany, Albany Publ., 1889, 595 pp.

Heitman, F. B.: *Historical Register and Dictionary of the United States Army.* Washington, Gov't. Printing Office, 2 vols., 1903.

Johnson, R. U., and Buel, C. C., Editors: *Battles and Leaders of the Civil War.* New York, Appleton, 4 vols., 1884-1888.

Medical and Surgical History of the War of the Rebellion (1861-65). Washington, Gov't. Printing Office, 6 vols., 1875-1888.

Military Order of the Loyal Legion of the United States. Obituaries and war papers published by the state commanderies under various titles, 1875-1915.

Miller, F. T., Editor: *Photographic History of the Civil War.* New York, Review of Reviews, 10 vols., 1911-12.

Moore, F., Editor: *Rebellion Record.* New York, Various publishers, 12 vols., 1861-1868.

National Archives: Military pension and military service files.

National Cyclopaedia of American Biography. New York, Appleton, 50 + vols., 1906 continuing to date (abbr. as "NCAB").

Phisterer, F.: *Statistical Record of the Armies of the United States.* New York, Scribner, 1883, 343 pp.

Regimental histories of the pertinent regiments, see C. E. Dornbusch: *Regimental Publications and Personal Narratives of the Civil War: A Checklist.* New York, New York Public Library, 1961 to date.

State military histories of the pertinent state.

Strait, N. A. (Revised): *An Alphabetical List and a Roster of all the Regimental Surgeons and Assistant Surgeons.* Washington, Van Buren, 1883, 330 pp.

Warner, E. J.: *Generals in Blue.* Baton Rouge, Louisiana State Univ. Press, 1964, 680 pp.

Warner, E. J.: *Generals in Gray.* Baton Rouge, Louisiana State Univ. Press, 1959, 330 pp.

War of the Rebellion: A Compilation of the Official Records of the Union and Confederate Armies. Washington, Gov't Printing Office, Four Series with 128 parts in 69 vols., 1880-1902 (abbr. as "O.R.").

B. Special References

Adams, G. W.: *Doctors in Blue.* New York, Schuman, 1952, 253 pp.

Anderson, A. F.: Death notice. *J. S. Carolina Med. Ass., 5*:559, 1909.

Anderson, J. P.: Autobiography of Gen. Patton Anderson, C.S.A. *So. Hist. Soc. Papers, 24*:57-72, 1896.

Anderson, J. Q: *A Texas Surgeon in the C.S.A.* Tuscaloosa, Confederate, 1957, 123 pp.

Andrews, Edmund.: *Complete Record of the Surgery of the Battles Fought Near Vicksburg, December 27, 28, 29, and 30, 1862.* Chicago, Fergus, 1863, 48 pp.

Andrews, E., and Woodworth, J. M.: *The Primary Surgery of Gen Sherman's Campaigns.* Chicago, Fergus, 1866, 20 pp.

Applegate, J. S.: *Reminiscences and Letters of George Arrowsmith of New Jersey.* Red Bank, Cook, 1893, 254 pp.

Aten, H. J.: *History of the Eighty-Fifth Regiment, Illinois Volunteer Infantry.* Hiawatha, Regimental Association, 1901, 506 pp.

Barney, C.: *Recollections of Field Service with the Twentieth Iowa Infantry Volunteers.* Davenport, Gazette Job Rooms, 1865, 323 pp.

Barry, A. R.: Obituary. *Confed. Vet. 11*:466, 1903.

Bassford, S. J.: Necrology, John E. L. Kimball, M.D., of Saco. *Trans. Maine Med. Ass., 11*:198, 1894.

Bates, S. P.: *History of the Pennsylvania Volunteers, 1861-5.* Harrisburg, Singerly, 5 vols., 1869-1871.

Bates, S. P.: *Martial Deeds of Pennsylvania.* Philadelphia, Davis, 1876, 1116 pp.

Baxter, J. H.: *Statistics, Medical and Anthropological, of the Provost-Marshal-General's Bureau.* Washington, Govt. Printing Office, 1875.

Beall, J. F.: Death notice. *Confed. Vet., 16,* 1908.

Billings, John: *Literature and Institutions, in A Century of American Medicine, 1776-1876.* by E. H. Clarke, *et al.* Philadelphia, Lea, 1876, 366 pp.

Blodgett, W. H.: Address on the occasion of the dedication of the monument, Brevet Major-General John McNeil. *Proc. of Frank P. Blair Post, No. 1, Dept. of Mo.,* G.A.R., 1894.

Blunt, J. G.: General Blunt's account of his Civil War experiences. *Kansas Hist. Quart., 1*:211-265, 1932.

Bourke, J. M.: *On the Border with Crook.* New York, Scribner, 1891.

Bowen, J. L.: *Massachusetts in the War, 1861-1865.* Springfield, Bryan, 1889, 1027 pp.

Bowen, J. R.: *Regimental History of the First New York Dragoons.* [No city], Published by the Author, 1900, 464 pp.

Brady, R.: *The Story of One Regiment: The Eleventh Maine Infantry Volunteers in the War of the Rebellion.* New York: J. J. Little, 1896, 435 pp.

Bratton, J.: The Sixth South Carolina at Seven Pines. *So. Hist. Soc. Papers, 13*:119-133, 1885.

Brown, F. H.: *Roll of Students of Harvard University Who Served in the Army or Navy of the United States During the War of the Rebellion.* Cambridge, Welch, Bigelow, 1866, 48 pp.

Brown, H. E.: Biography. *Med. News, 55*:213, 1889.

Brown, H. E.: *The Medical Department of the United States Army from 1775 to 1873.* Washington, Surgeon-General's Office, 1873, 314 pp.

Brown, J. W.: *The Signal Corps, U.S.A. in the War of the Rebellion.* Boston, U.S. Vet. Signal Corps Assoc., 1896, pp. 916.

Brown, O.: Death notice. *J.A.M.A., 43*:558, 1904.

Brown, O.: In memoriam, Orlando Brown, Brevet Brigadier General, U. S. Volunteers. *Commandery of the State of New York, Military Order of the Loyal Legion,* Circular No. 33, Series of 1904.

Butler, B. F.: *Butler's Book: Autobiography and Personal Reminiscences of Major-General Benj. F. Butler.* Boston, Thayer, 1892, 1154 pp.

Byers, S. H. M.: *Iowa in War Times.* Des Moines, Condit, 1888, 615 pp.

Capehart, H.: Record No. 10774, Military Order of the Loyal Legion of the U.S.

Castel, A.: *A Frontier State at War: Kansas, 1861-1865.* Ithaca, Cornell Univ. Press, 1958, 251 pp.

Chase, J. J.: *The Charge at Daybreak: Scenes and Incidents at the Battle of the Mine Explosion, Near Petersburg, Virginia.* Lewiston, Journal Office, 1875, 32 pp.

Clark, W.: *Histories of Several Regiments and Battalions From North Carolina in the Great War 1861-65.* Goldsboro, Nash Bros., Vol. 2, 1901.

Cogley, T. S.: *History of the Seventh Indiana Cavalry Volunteers.* Laporte, Herald, 1876, 267 pp.

Coolidge, R. H.: Report with regard to the removal of the wounded after the second battle of Manassas. *Medical and Surgical History of the War of the Rebellion:* Part I, Vol. I, Appendix page 124-126.

Corner, G. W.: *The Autobiography of Benjamin Rush.* Princeton, Princeton Univ. Press, 1948, 399 pp.

Crawford, S. W.: University of Pennsylvania, *Archives and Records Center.*

Crawford, S. W.: An essay on hypertrophy and atrophy. Thesis for the Degree of Doctor of Medicine, University of Pennsylvania, Feb. 4, 1850. Manuscript, 19 pp.

Crawford, S. W.: *The Genesis of the Civil War.* New York, Webster, 1887.

Crawford, S. W.: *Papers of Samuel W. Crawford.* Library of Congress, Manuscript Division.

Croffut, W. A., and Morris, J. M.: *The Military and Civil History of Connecticut During the War of 1861-65,* 3rd ed. New York, Ledyard Bill., 1869, 891 pp.

Cudworth, W. H.: *History of the First Regiment (Massachusetts Infantry).* Boston, Walker, Fuller, 1866, 528 pp.

Cunningham, H. H.: *Doctors in Gray: The Confederate Medical Service.* Baton Rouge, Louisiana State Univ. Press, 1958, 339 pp.

Curtis, N. M.: *From Bull Run to Chancellorsville.* New York, Putnam, 1906, 384 pp.

Dana, C. A.: *Recollections of the Civil War.* New York, Appleton, 1902, 296 pp.

Davenport, A.: *Camp and Field of the Fifth New York Volunteer Infantry (Duryee Zouaves).* New York, Dick & Fitzgerald, 1879, 485 pp.

Davenport, E. A.: *History of the Ninth Regiment Illinois Cavalry Volunteers.* Chicago, Historical Committee, 1888, 448 pp.

Delong, I. F.: Report of Col. J. W. Robertson, Thirty-fifth Regiment Alabama Volunteers. *O.R., 15*:96.

Dickert, D. A.: *History of Kershaw's Brigade.* Newberry, Hull, 1899, 583 pp.

Doubleday, A.: *Reminiscences of Forts Sumter and Moultrie in 1860-1861.* New York, Harper, 1876, 184 pp.

Dowley, M. F.: *History and Honorary Roll of the Twelfth Regiment, Infantry, N. G. S. N. Y.* New York, Farrell, 1869, 216 pp.

Duffee, W. G.: *In the Biographical Encyclopedia of Pennsylvania of the Nineteenth Century.* Philadelphia, Galaxy, 1874, 672 pp.

Duke, B. W.: *Reminiscences of General Basil W. Duke, C.S.A.* Garden City, Doubleday, 1911, 512 pp.

Duncan, L. C.: *The Medical Department of the United States Army in the Civil War.* Washington, various pagination, reprinted from *Military Medicine,* 1914.

Dustin, D.: In Memoriam, Col. and Brevet Brigadier General Daniel Dustin. *Commandery of the State of Illinois, Military Order of the Loyal Legion.* Circular No. 9, Series of 1892.

Eddy, T. M.: *The Patriotism of Illinois.* Chicago, Clarke, 2 vols. 1865-66.

Elliott, I. H., and Way, V. G.: *History of the Thirty-Third Regiment Illinois Veteran Volunteer Infantry.* Gibson City, Publ. by the Association, 1902, 288 pp.

Elliott, S. M.: Obituary. *Commandery of the State of New York, Military Order of the Loyal Legion.* Circular No. 5, Series of 1875-76.

Ellis, T. T.: *Leaves from the Diary of an Army Surgeon.* New York, Bradburn, 1863, 312 pp.

Elwell, J. J.: *Medical Jurisprudence: A Medico-legal Treatise on Malpractice and Medical Evidence.* New York, Voorhies, 1860, 588 pp.

Ely, J. F.: *First Year's Medical History of the Twenty-Fourth Iowa. In "War Sketches and Incidents."* Iowa Commandery, Military Order of the Loyal Legion. Des Moines, Kenyon, Vol. 1, 1893, 400 pp.

Ewer, J. K.: *The Third Massachusetts Cavalry in the War for the Union.* Hist. Comm. of the Regimental Association, 1903, 452 pp.

Fishbein, M.: *A History of the American Medical Association, 1847 to 1947.* Philadelphia and London, Saunders, 1947, 1226 pp.

Foster, J. Y.: *New Jersey and the Rebellion.* Newark, Dennis, 1868, 872 pp.

Fox, W. B.: *What I Remember of the Great Rebellion.* Lansing, Thorpe, 1892, 278 pp.

Gano, R. M.: Death notice. *J. A. M. A., 60*:1170, 1913.

Gano, R. M.: Biography in *Handbook of Texas.* Texas Hist. Assn., Vol. 2, 1952.

Gibbon, J.: *Personal Recollections of the Civil War.* New York, Putnam, 1928, 426 pp.

Gleason, D. H. L.: *A History of the First Regiment of Massachusetts Cavalry Volunteers.* Boston, Houghton, 1891, 490 pp.

Gordon, G. H.: *A War Diary of Events in the War of the Great Rebellion, 1863-1865.* Boston, Osgood, 1882, 437 pp.

Gordon, S. C.: Reminiscences of the Civil War from a surgeon's point of view. In *War Papers.* Maine Commandery, Military Order of the Loyal Legion. Portland, (no publisher), Vol. 1, 1898.

Gorgas, J.: Ordnance of the Confederacy. *So. His. Soc. Papers, 12*:67-94, 1884.

Gunn, M.: *Memorial Sketches of Doctor Moses Gunn, by His Wife.* Chicago, Keener, 1889, 380 pp.

Hall, C. R.: The lessons of the War Between the States. *Int. Rec. Med., 171*:408-430, 1958.

Hancock, P. R.: *Hancock's Diary: or, A History of the Second Tennessee Confederate Cavalry.* Nashville, Brandon, 1887, 644 pp.

Hard, A.: *History of the Eighth Cavalry Regiment Illinois Volunteers, During The Great Rebellion.* Aurora (no publisher), 1868, 368 pp.

Harris, T. M.: *Assassination of Lincoln.* Boston, American Citizen, 1892, 424 pp.

Harrison, E. B.: Eugene Beauharnais Harrison, M.D. *J.A.M.A., 46*:1305, 1906.

Harrison, E. B.: Death: Dr. Eugene B. Harrison, *Ohio Med. J. 1*:550, 1906.

Hart, A. G.: The surgeon and the hospital in the Civil War. Papers, *Mil. Hist. Soc. Mass., 13*:229-285, 1902.

Hart, E. J.: *History of the Fortieth Illinois Infantry Volunteers.* Cincinnati, Bosworth, 1864, 197 pp.

Haskell, J. C.: *The Haskell Memoirs.* edited by G. E. Govan, and J. W. Livingood. New York, Putnam, 1960, 176 pp.

Hassler, W. W.: *A. P. Hill: Lee's Forgotten General.* Richmond, Garrett & Massie, 1957, 249 pp.

Hay, T. R.: Lucius B. Northrop: Commissary General of the Confederacy. *Civil War History, 9*:5-23, 1963.

Headley, P. C.: *Massachusetts in the Rebellion.* Boston, Walker, Fuller, 1866, 688 pp.

Henry, R. S.: *"First With the Most" Forrest.* Indianapolis, Bobbs-Merrill, 1944, 558 pp.

Hewitt, S. M.: *O.R., 19*:566-576.

Hill, J. A.: *The Story of One Regiment.* New York, Little, 1896, 435 pp.

Hillis, D. B.: Obituary. *J.A.M.A., 35*:836, 1900.

Historical Committee. *A History of the Seventy-Third Regiment of Illinois Infantry Volunteers.* Regimental Reunion Assn. of Survivors, 1890, 682 pp.

Houston, H. C.: *The Thirty-Second Maine Regiment of Infantry Volunteers.* Portland, Southworth 1903, 537 pp.

Howard, R. L.: *History of the One Hundred Twenty-fourth Regiment Illinois Infantry Volunteers.* Springfield, Rokker, 1880, 519 pp.

Hume, E. E.: *Ornithologists of the United States Army Medical Corps.* Baltimore, Johns Hopkins 1942, 581 pp.

Hurd, A.: Anson Hurd, M.D. *J.A.M.A., 54*:900, 1910.

Illinois, Report of the Adjutant General of the State of. Springfield, Rokker, 8 vols., Revised, 1886.

Indiana, Report of the Adjutant General of the State of, 1861-1865. Indianapolis, Holloway, 1865.

The Soldier of Indiana in the War for the Union. Indianapolis, Merrill, 2 vols., 1866, 1869.

Ingersoll, L. D.: *Iowa and the Rebellion.* 3rd Ed. Philadelphia, Lippincott, 1867, 743 pp.

Iowa, Report of the Adjutant General and the Acting Quartermaster General of. Des Moines, Palmer, 2 vols., 1863.

Johnson, J. L.: *The University Memorial: Biographical Sketches of Alumni of the University of Virginia Who Fell in the Confederate War.* Baltimore, Turnbull, 1871, 765 pp.

Jones, J.: Roster of the medical officers of the Army of Tennessee. *So. Hist. Soc. Papers, 22*:165-280, 1894.

Jones, J. C.: The death of Dr. John C. Jones. *Texas Med. News, 13*:252, 1903-1904.

Jones, J. C.: Biography. *So. Hist. Soc. Papers, 22*:221-223, 1894.

Kelly, H. A.: *A Cyclopedia of American Medical Biography.* Chicago, Saunders, 1912.

Kansas, Report of the Adjutant General of the State of: Leavenworth, Bulletin Co-Operative Printing, Vol. I, 1867.

Keene, F. E.: George H. Lyman, M.D.: In *Album of the Fellows of the American Gynecological Society, 1876-1930.* Philadelphia, Dorman, 1930, 640 pp.

Kemper, G. W. H.: *A Medical History of the State of Indiana.* Chicago, A.M.A. Press, 1911, 393 pp.

Kemper, W. H.: The Surgeons of the Civil War. *J. Indiana Med. Ass., 11*:367-369, 1918.

Kepler, W.: *History of the Fourth Regiment Ohio Volunteer Infantry.* Cleveland, Leader, 1886, 287 pp.

Kimball, N.: In Memoriam. *Commandery of the State of Nebraska, Military Order of the Loyal Legion.* Circular No. 4, Series of 1898.

King, C.: Rufus King: Soldier, editor, and statesman. *Wisconsin Magazine of History, 4*: No. 4, June, 1921, 13 pp.

Lang, T. F.: *Loyal West Virginia from 1861 to 1865.* Baltimore, Deutsch, 1895, 382 pp.

Leasure, D.: *Personal Observations and Experiences in the Pope Campaign in Virginia.* In: *Glimpses of the Nation's Struggle.* Vol. 1, St. Paul, St. Paul, 1887, 135-166.

Leasure, D.: The erysipelatous disease of lying-in women. *Amer. J. Med. Sci., 31*:45-49, 1856.

Leggett, M. D.: In Memoriam. *Commandery of the State of Ohio, Military Order of the Loyal Legion.* Circular No. 8, Series of 1896.

Lewis, G. R.: Biography. *Confed. Vet., 21*:401, 1913.

Lewis, J. M.: War papers. *Wisconsin Commandery of the Military Order of the Loyal Legion,* Vol. 1, 1891, 132.

Lewis, S. E.: Dr. Samuel P. Moore: The Surgeon-General of the Confederate States. *So. Hist. Soc. Papers, 29*:273-279, 1901.

Lippitt, F. J.: *Reminiscences of Francis J. Lippitt.* Providence, Preston & Rounds, 1902, 122 pp.

Livermore, T. L.: *Days and Events, 1860-1866.* Boston and New York, Houghton, 1920, 420 pp.

Lloyd, F.: General Alexander Chambers. *Iowa. Hist. Record, 9*:385-393, 1893.

Logan, J. A.: *The Volunteer Soldier of America.* Chicago and New York, Peale, 1887, 706 pp.

Logan, J. A.: *The Great Conspiracy: Its Origin and History.* New York, Hart, 1886, 810 pp.

Logan, Mrs. J. A.: *Reminiscences of a Soldier's Wife, an Autobiography.* New York, Scribner, 1916, 470 pp.

Ludlow, B. C.: Necrology. *J.A.M.A., 30*:334, 1898.

Lyman, G. H.: *Non-Malignant Diseases of the Uterus.* Boston, Ticknor & Fields, 1854, 76 pp.

Lyman, G. H.: Necrology. *J.A.M.A., 17*:387, 1891.

Lyman, G. H.: Some aspects of the medical service in the armies of the United States during the War of the Rebellion. Papers, *Milit. Hist. Soc. Mass., 13*:175-228, 1913.

Magee, B. F.: *History of the Seventy-second Indiana Volunteer Infantry.* LaFayette, Vater, 1882, 698 pp.

Maine, Annual Report of the Adjutant General of the State of. Augusta, Stevens & Sayward, 1863.

Mangrum, L. H.: In *Campaigns and Battles of the Sixteenth Regiment Tennessee Volunteers.* by T. A. Head. Nashville, Cumberland, 1885, 488 pp.

Marshall, P.: *A Life of William B. Bate, Citizen, Soldier and Statesman.* Nashville, Cumberland, 1908, 363 pp.

Martin, J. M., *et al.*: *History of the Fifty-Seventh Regiment, Pennsylvania Veteran Volunteer Infantry.* Meadville, McCoy and Calvin, 1904, 196 pp.

Martin, R. W.: Biography. *Confed. Vet., 5*:70, 1897.

Massachusetts, Annual Report of the Adjutant General of the Commonwealth of. Boston, Wright & Potter, 1865.

Massachusetts, Record of Massachusetts Volunteers, 1861-1865. Boston, Wright & Potter, 2 vols., 1868, 1870.

Massachusetts. History of the Thirty-Fifth Regiment Massachusetts Volunteers, 1862-1865. by a Committee of the Regimental Assn. Boston, Mills, Knight, 1884, 409 pp.

Matheny, H. E.: *Major General Thomas Maley Harris.* Parsons, McClain, 1963, 296 pp.

Maxwell, J. D.: Biography of John G. McPheeters. *Trans. Indiana State Med. Assn.,* 1888, 212 pp.

McAdams, F. M.: *Every-Day Soldier Life, or A History of the One Hundred and Thirteenth Ohio Volunteer Infantry.* Columbus, Cott, 1884, 400 pp.

McGugin, D. L.: *In One Hundred Years of Iowa Medicine.* Iowa City, Athens 1950, 483.

McGugin, D. L.: Extracts from a report on the operations of the medical department during the battle of Pea Ridge. *Medical and Surgical History of the War of the Rebellion,* Part I, Vol. I, Appendix 340-341.

McGuire, H.: Biography. *Confed. Vet., 8*:411-412, 1900.

McLaughlin, J. M.: Biography. *Confed. Vet., 17*:174, 1909.

McMillen, W. L.: In Memoriam. *Ohio Commandery, Military Order of the Loyal Legion.* Circular No. 18, Series of 1902.

McMurry, J. W.: *History of the Twentieth Tennessee Volunteer Infantry, C.S.A.* Nashville, Publication Committee, 1904, 520 pp.

Meeker, D.: *Opium Eating, Its Consequences and Cure.* Laporte, 1872-73.

Memorandum Relative to the General Officers Appointed by the Presi-

dent in the Armies of the Confederate States, 1861-1865. Washington, Govt. Printing Office, 1908, 41 pp.

Memorandum Relative to the General Officers in the Armies of the United States During the Civil War, 1861-1865. Washington, Govt. Printing Office, 1908, 73 pp.

Merchant, T. E.: *Eighty-Fourth Regiment, Pennsylvania Volunteers (Infantry).* Philadelphia, Sherman, 109 pp.

Merritt, W.: *A Century of Medicine in Jacksonville and Duval County.* Gainesville, Univ. of Florida Press, 1949, 201 pp.

Milhau, J. J.: Obituary. *Med. Rec., 39*:576, 1891.

Missouri, Annual Report of the Adjutant General of. Jefferson City, Foster, 1868, 781 pp.

Moore, S. P.: Obituary. *Virginia Med. Monthly, 16*:250-254, 1889-1890.

Mulligan, J. A.: In *Battles and Leaders, 1*:307.

Myer, A. J.: *A New Sign Language for Deaf Mutes.* Buffalo, Jewett, Thomas, 1851, 12 pp.

Myer, A. J.: *Manual of Signals.* New York, Van Nostrand, New ed., 1866, 398 pp.

Newhaus, C.: *Medical and Surgical History of the War of the Rebellion,* Part II, Vol. II, 474, 488.

Newman, A.: Albert Newman, M.D. *J.A.M.A., 44*:1549, 1905.

Newman, A.: *Comparison of the Mortality from Diseases in Armies.* Leavenworth, Times & Conservative Printing, 1869, 39 pp.

Nichols, G. W.: *The Story of the Great March.* New York, Harper, 1865, 408 pp.

Nicolay, J. G., and Hay, J.: *Abraham Lincoln: A History.* New York, Appleton, Vol. 5, 141.

Niles, J. M.: *The Life of Oliver Hazard Perry, and a View of the Leading Events in the Life of General Harrison.* 2nd ed., Hartford, Cooke, 1821, 384 pp.

Oates, W. C.: *The War Between the Union and the Confederacy, With a History of the Fifteenth Alabama Regiment.* New York and Washington, Neale, 1905, 808 pp.

Ohio Roster Commission. *Official Roster of the Soldiers of the State of Ohio in the War of the Rebellion, 1861-1866.* Akron, Authority of the General Assembly, 11 vols., 1886-1891.

Orton, R. H.: *Records of California Men in the War of the Rebellion, 1861 to 1867.* Sacramento, Young, 1890, 887 pp.

Osborne, W. A.: *History of the Twenty-Ninth Regiment of Massachusetts Volunteer Infantry.* Boston, Wright, 1877, 393 pp.

Owens, T. M.: Philip Dale Roddy, *in History of Alabama and Dictionary of Alabama Biography.* Chicago, Clarke, 1921, Vol. 4, 1454-1455.

Palmer, T. M.: *Palmer Doctors.* Unpublished typescript.

Park, R. E.: *Sketch of the Twelfth Alabama Infantry.* Richmond, Jones, 1906, 106 pp.

Parker, F. J.: *Story of the Thirty-Second Regiment Massachusetts Infantry.* Boston, Calkins, 1880, 260 pp.

Partridge, C. A.: *History of the Ninety-Sixth Regiment Illinois Volunteer Infantry.* Chicago, Hist. Soc. of the Regiment, 1887, 938 pp.

Payne, E. W.: *History of the Thirty-Fourth Regiment of Illinois Infantry.* Clinton, Allen, 1902, 370 pp.

Phisterer, F.: *Statistical Record of the Armies of the United States.* New York, Scribner, 1883, 343 pp.

Phisterer, F.: *New York in the War of the Rebellion, 1861 to 1865.* 3rd Ed. Albany, Lyon, 5 vols. and Index, 1912.

Pollard, E. A.: *Lee and His Lieutenants.* New York, Treat, 1867, 851 pp.

Powell, W. H.: *Officers of the Army and Navy (Volunteer) Who Served in the Civil War.* Philadelphia, Hamersly, 1893, 419 pp.

Reader, F. S.: *History of the Fifth West Virginia Cavalry.* New Brighton, Daily News, 1890, 304 pp.

Reid, W.: *Ohio in the War.* Cincinnati, Moore, Wilstack & Baldwin, 1868, 2 vols.

Rerick, J. H.: *Forty-Fourth Indiana Volunteer Infantry.* La Grange, Publ. by the Author, 1880, 293 pp.

Riley, H. D.: Medicine in the Confederacy. *Milit. Med., 118*:53-63, 114-153, 1956.

Robertson, J.: *Michigan in the War.* Lansing, George, Revised ed., 1882, 1039 pp.

Roe, A. S., and Nutt, C.: *History of the First Regiment of Heavy Artillery Massachusetts Volunteers.* Worcester and Boston, Regimental Association, 1917, 507 pp.

Russo, D. R.: *One Hundred Years of Indiana Medicine, 1849-1949.* Cent. Ind. State Med. Ass., 1949, 195 pp.

Satchwell, S. C.: Medico-chirurgical lessons of the late war from Southern standpoints. *Virginia Med. Monthly, 1*:35-37, 1874.

Schmitt, M. E.: *General George Crook, His Autobiography.* Norman, Univ. of Oklahoma Press, 1946, 326 pp.

Schouler, W.: *A History of Massachusetts in the Civil War.* Boston, Dutton, 2 vols., 1868, 1871.

Scott, J. J.: Biography. *Confed. Vet., 16*:86, 1908.

Scott, W. F.: *Story of a Cavalry Regiment, Fourth Iowa.* New York, Putnam, 1893, 602 pp.

Shastid, T. H.: A short biography of Dr. John J. Elwell. *Amer. Med., 4*:94-96, 1909.

Shaw, J. B.: *History of the Tenth Regiment Indiana Volunteer Infantry.* Lafayette (no publisher), 1912, 325 pp.

Sherman, W. T.: *Memoirs of Gen. W. T. Sherman.* 4th ed., New York, Webster, 2 vols., 1891.

Sipes, W. B.: *Seventh Pennsylvania Veteran Volunteer Cavalry.* Pottsville, Miner's Journal, 1905, 169 plus 60 plus 142.

Smith, A. P.: *History of the Seventy-Sixth Regiment New York Volunteers.* Cortland, by the Author, 1867, 429 pp.

Smith, D. P.: *Medical and Surgical History of the War of the Rebellion,* Part I, Vol. I, Appendix p. 24.

Smith, D. P.: Obituary. *Boston Med. Surg. J., 103*:646, 1880.

Speer, A. M.: Obituary. *J.A.M.A., 65*:546, 1915.

Stedman, C. E.: In Memoriam, George Hinckley Lyman. *Boston Med. Surg. J., 126*:313-318, 1892.

Stark, R. B.: Surgeons and surgical care of the Confederate States Army. *Virginia Med. Monthly, 87*:230-241, 1960.

Steiner, P. E.: *Medical Military Portraits of Union and Confederate Generals.* In preparation.

Steiner, P. E.: Medical military studies on the Civil War: I. Lieutenant General Ambrose Powell Hill, C.S.A. *Milit. Med., 130*:225-228, 1965.

Stevens, H.: *Life of Isaac Ingalls Stevens by His Son, Hazard Stevens.* Boston and New York, Houghton, 2 vols., 1901.

Stevenson, T. M.: *History of the Seventy-Eighth Regiment O. V. V. I.* Zanesville, Dunne, 1865, 349 pp.

Stewart, N. B.: *Dan McCook's Regiment, Fifty-Second O. V. I.* Alliance, By the Author, 1900, 225 pp.

Stone, J. M.: Dr. John E. L. Kimball. *In: History of the Twenty-Seventh Regiment Maine Volunteer Infantry.* Portland, Thurston Press, 1895, 44 pp.

Stone, R. F.: *Biography of Eminent American Physicians and Surgeons.* Indianapolis, Carlon & Hollenbeck, 1894, 729 pp.

Stowits, G. H.: *History of the One Hundredth Regiment of New York State Volunteers.* Buffalo, Matthew & Warren, 1870, 424 pp.

Stryker, W. S.: *Record of Officers and Men of New Jersey in the Civil War, 1861-1865.* Trenton, Murphy, 2 vols., 1876.

Stuart, A. A.: *Iowa Colonels and Regiments.* Des Moines, Mills, 1865, 656 pp.

Sutton, J. J.: *History of the Second Regiment West Virginia Cavalry Volunteers.* Portsmouth (no publisher), 1892, 262 pp.

Sypher, J. R.: *History of the Pennsylvania Reserve Corps.* Lancaster Barr, 1865, 723 pp.

Rawling, C. J.: *History of the First Regiment Virginia Infantry.* Philadelphia, Lippincott, 1887, 284 pp.

Thomas, H. W.: *History of the Doles-Cook Brigade Army of Northern Virginia, C.S.A.* Atlanta, Franklin, 1903, 632 pp.

Thrall, S. B.: An Iowa doctor in blue: The letters of Seneca B. Thrall, 1862-1864. Ed. by M. Throne. *Iowa J. Hist., 58*:97-188, 1960.

Todd, W.: *Seventy-Ninth Highlanders New York Volunteers in the War of the Rebellion, 1861-1865.* Albany, Brandon, Barton, 1886, 513 pp.

Toner, J. M.: *Medical Men of the American Revolution.* Philadelphia, Collins, 1876, 140 pp.

Toombs, S.: *New Jersey Troops in the Gettysburg Campaign from June 5 to July 31, 1863.* Orange, Evening Mail, 1888, 406 pp.

Vandiver, F. E.: *Civil War Diary of General Josiah Gorgas.* University, Univ. of Alabama Press, 1947, 208 pp.

University of Pennsylvania, Archives and Records Center.

Wailes, L. A.: A case of field surgery. *Confed. Vet., 25*:107, 1917.

Waite, F. C.: *Western Reserve University, Centennial History of the School of Medicine.* Cleveland, Western Reserve U. Press, 1946, 588 pp.

Waitt, E. L.: *History of the Nineteenth Regiment Massachusetts Volunteer Infantry.* Salem, Salem Press, 1906, 446 pp.

Walcott, C. F.: *History of the Twenty-First Regiment Massachusetts Volunteers.* Boston, Houghton, 1882, 502 pp.

Warner, L. F.: Obituary of David Paige Smith. *Trans. Amer. Med. Ass., 32*:539, 1881.

Ware, E. F.: *The Lyon Campaign in Missouri.* Topeka, Crane, 1907, 377 pp.

Washburn, G. H.: *Military History and Record of the One Hundred and Eighth Regiment New York Volunteers.* Rochester, Andrews, 1894, 521 pp.

Wentworth, M. F.: In memoriam. *Maine Commandery, Military Order of the Loyal Legion.* Circular No. 7, Series of 1897.

West Virginia, Annual Report of the Adjutant General of. Wheeling, John Frew, 1866, 444 p.

Weygant, C. H.: *History of the One hundred and Twenty-Fourth Regiment, N. Y. S. V.* Newburgh, Journal Printing House, 1877, 460 pp.

Whitman, W. E. S., and True, C. H.: *Maine in the War for the Union.* Lewiston, Dingley, 1865, 592 pp.

Wickham, J. P.: Surgical department of the Confederate Army: Samuel Preston Moore, Surgeon General, C.S.A. *Confed. Vet., 33*:406-407, 1925.

Wild, E.: Necrology, *J.A.M.A., 17*:702, 1891.

Wild, E. A.: *Medical and Surgical History of the War of the Rebellion,* Part II, Volume II, p. 629.

Willard, J. N.: *History of the Nineteenth Regiment Massachusetts Volunteer Infantry.* Salem, Historical Committee, 1906, 456 pp.

Wilson, J. G.: *Biographical Sketches of Illinois Officers Engaged in the War.* Chicago, Barnet, 1862, 104 pp.

Wilson, J. H.: *Under the Old Flag.* New York and London, Appleton, 2 vols. 1912.

Wood, C. J.: *Reminiscences of the War.* (No city, no publisher, no date), 283 pp.

Woodhull, A. A.: An inquiry into the military rights and duties of medical officers in the land forces. *U. S. Service Magazine, 1*:478-489, 1864.

Woodhull, A. A.: Eligibility of medical officers of the army as members of certain courts-martial. *U. S. Service Magazine, 1*:258-263, 1864.

Wyeth, J. A.: *That Devil Forest: Life of General Nathan Bedford Forrest.* New York, Harper, 1959, 614 pp.

C. References to the Official Records

(Note: "O.R." refers to the *War of the Rebellion: A Compilation of the Official Records of the Union and Confederate Armies.* Washington: Gov't. Printing Office, 1880-1902, published in four series with sixty-nine volumes containing 128 parts (i.e., separate books). Unless otherwise specified the reference is to Series I.)

1. O.R., *38:* part 3, 109, 200, 696, 769-775.
2. O.R., *47:* part 1, 808.
3. O.R., Index volume.
4. O.R., *52:* part 2, 598-599.
5. O.R., 22: part 1, 84-85.
6. O.R., *41:* part 1, 571-581.
7. O.R., *22:* part 2, 398-399, 465-466.
8. O.R., *53:* 565-567, 571-573.
9. O.R., *34:* part 3, 133.
10. O.R., *34:* part 1, 790-791.

11. O.R., *22:* part 2, 465-466.
12. O.R., *11:* part 2, 672, 751, 755.
13. O.R., Series IV, *2:* 923.
14. O.R., *39:* part 2, 724.
15. O.R., *49:* part 1, 829, 937.
16. O.R., *42:* part 1, 875-876.
17. O.R., *11:* part 1, 858-859, 890, 896, 947-948.
18. O.R., *42:* part 1, 878-883.
19. O.R., Series III, *3:* 1143.
20. O.R., *46:* part 3, 1170.
21. O.R., *8:* 207.
22. O.R., *41:* part 1, 976.
23. O.R., *48:* part 1, 1216.
24. O.R., *22:* part 2, 53.
25. O.R., *34:* part 1, 259.
26. O.R., *34:* part 4, 616.
27. O.R., *27:* part 1, 995 and part 2, 123, 388.
28. O.R., *43:* part 1, 510.
29. O.R., *46:* part 1, 475-476, 482, 1111.
30. O.R., *47:* part 3, 56, 96.
31. O.R., *38:* part 1, 106.
32. O.R., *38:* part 3, 283.
33. O.R., *30:* part 1, 177, 858, 861, 863.
34. O.R., *23:* part 2, 579.
35. O.R., *38:* part 1, 226, 244-245.
36. O.R., *19:* part 1, 474-478, 484-486.
37. O.R., *39:* part 1, 679-682, 687.
38. O.R., *14:* 50.
39. O.R., *53:* 80.
40. O.R., *14:* 394.
41. O.R., *28:* part 2, 4, 18, 104.
42. O.R., Series III, *5:* 348.
43. O.R., *26:* part 2, 121.
44. O.R., *22:* part 1, 34 and part 2, 1048.
45. O.R., *34:* part 2, 874.
46. O.R., *53:* 964.
47. O.R., *34:* part 1, 783 and part 3, 826.
48. O.R., *34:* part 2, 874.
49. O.R., *12:* part 1, 5.
50. O.R., *19:* part 2, 338, 370, 522.

51. O.R., *25:* part 2, 34, 134, 591.
52. O.R., *27:* part 2, 209-210.
53. O.R., *33:* 976.
54. O.R., *43:* part 1, 115, 123, 134, 371-374.
55. O.R., *43:* part 1, 3901391.
56. O.R., *46:* part 1, 129.
57. O.R., *24:* part 1, 777.
58. O.R., *26:* part 1, 712.
59. O.R., Series III, *3:* 740.
60. O.R., *5:* 186-187, 221-222.
61. O.R., *11:* part 2, 922.
62. O.R., *12:* part 1, 360-361.
63. O.R., *21:* 262.
64. O.R., *19:* part 1, 324.
65. O.R., *19:* part 1, 173, 193, 326-328.
66. O.R., *21:* 131, 286, 289-291.
67. O.R., *52:* part 1, 336, 341.
68. O.R., *24:* part 2, 436-438.
69. O.R., *24:* 359, 364, 366, 369, 379, 576.
70. O.R., *22:* part 2, 394, 395, 407, 453, 530, 585.
71. O.R., *22:* part 2, 709.
72. O.R., *31:* part 3, 360.
73. O.R., *32:* part 2, 42, 190.
74. O.R., *34:* part 2, 225.
75. O.R., Series III, *3:* 1156.
76. O.R., *34:* part 2, 646-647.
77. O.R., *34:* part 3, 694, 704-705.
78. O.R., *34:* part 3, 132, 255-257, 280, 299.
79. O.R., *38:* part 5, 802.
80. O.R., *45:* part 1, 177-183.
81. O.R., *45:* part 2, 542.
82. O.R., *48:* part 2, 1042, 1061, 1167.
83. O.R., *12:* part 1, 344-345.
84. O.R., *24:* part 2, 565.
85. O.R., *47:* part 2, 42.
86. O.R., *38:* part 3, 20.
87. O.R., *38:* part 3, 555.
88. O.R., *7:* 633, 654.
89. O.R., *24:* part 1, 647.
90. O.R., *38:* part 5, 634.

91. O.R., *47:* part 1, 207.
92. O.R., *24:* part 2, 151.
93. O.R., *24:* part 1, 618.
94. O.R., *27:* part 2, 786.
95. O.R., *29:* part 1, 16, 246.
96. O.R., *40:* part 2, 60, 531, and part 3, 268, 491, 676.
97. O.R., *36:* part 2, 798.
98. O.R., *42:* part 1, 650, and part 2, 101, 107, 181, 232.
99. O.R., *42:* part 3, 98, 351, 783, 896.
100. O.R., *46:* part 2, 472, 682, 753.
101. O.R., *46:* part 3, 567, 569, 739, 985.
102. O.R., *16:* part 1, 914, 922, 928-930.
103. O.R., *24:* part 1, 762, 766.
104. O.R., *39:* part 1, 103-106, 206.
105. O.R., *39:* part 1, 258-261.
106. O.R., *42:* part 2, 210, 235.
107. O.R., *7:* 86, 92.
108. O.R., *30:* part 1, 449-453, 463-466.
109. O.R., *49:* part 1, 361, 446-449.
110. O.R., *31:* part 1, 466-470.
111. O.R., *29:* part 2, 869-870.
112. O.R., *34:* part 4, 692.
113. O.R., *41:* part 3, 917.
114. O.R., *48:* part 2, 1281, 1291, 1296.
115. O.R., *11:* part 2, 564, 569.
116. O.R., *12:* part 2, 606, 617-619.
117. O.R., *27:* part 2, 404-407.
118. O.R., *17:* part 1, 333.
119. O.R., *38:* part 1, 109.
120. O.R., *44:* 803.
121. O.R., *12:* part 2, 369.
122. O.R., *19:* part 1, 170, 222, 234, 237.
123. O.R., Series III, *5:* 900.
124. O.R., *19:* part 1, 448.
125. O.R., *18:* 659, 723.
126. O.R., *28:* part 2, 30, 75.
127. O.R., *29:* part 2, 619.
128. O.R., *29:* part 1, 910-918.
129. O.R., *29:* part 2, 542, 562, 595, 597.
130. O.R., *46:* part 2, 679.

131. O.R., *40:* part 2, 202.
132. O.R., *47:* part 3, 604.
133. O.R., Series II, *6:* 776-777, 845-847.
134. O.R., *12:* part 2, 623.
135. O.R., *31:* part 2, 431.
136. O.R., *38:* part 2, 311.
137. O.R., *47:* part 1, 776.
138. O.R., *17:* part 2, 571
139. O.R., *10:* part 2, 57, 73.
140. O.R., Series III, *5:* 137.
141. O.R., *19:* part 1, 566-576.

INDEX

A

Additional professions or occupations, 108, 144-145
Age at enlistment, 122-123
  Gray-Beard regiment, 123
Allen, Surg. J. S., 12, 126, 142
Ambition for military distinction, 147, 160-161
Anderson, Surg. A. F., 12, 117
Anderson, Gen. J. P., 8, 10, 15-17, 72
Andrew, Gov. J. A., 100
Andrews, Surg. E., 136, 157

B

Barnes, Surg. Gen. J. K., 5
Bate, Gen. W. B., 8, 9, 110, 121, 122, 128, 130
Birth of physician-generals, date and place, 105, 112
Black, Lt. Col. H. H., 11, 119, 126, 128
Blenker, Gen. L., 6
Blunt, Gen. J. G., 17-21, 51, 63
Booth, Capt. L. F., 11, 118
Boyhood, rural *versus* urban, 105
Brady, Gen. T. J., 11, 144
Branch, Gen. L. O'B., 9, 110, 119, 122, 126, 127
Brandon, Gen. W. L., 8, 21-22
Bratton, Gen. J., 22-23
Brevard, Gen. T. W., 9, 110, 119
Bronchiectasis, chronic, 78
Brooks, Gen. W. T. H., 9, 113, 121, 126, 130, 133
Brown, Surg. H. E., 11, 141, 144
Brown, Col. J. M., 7
Brown, Gen. O., 24-26
Brown, Gen. P. P., 9
Brown, Col. W. N., 11
Buchanan, President James, 15
Burris, Col. J. T., 11
Bussey, Gen. C., 26-28, 74
Butler, Gen. Ben, 77, 125, 150
Byrne, Gen. J. J., 9, 121, 137

C

Caldwell, Gen. J. C., 9, 121, 133
Cameron, Gen. R. A., 8, 28-32
Cameron, Secretary S., 66
Capehart, Gen. H., 32-35
Captain Perrin's Company, 4
Carr, Gen. J. B., 9, 121, 125, 133, 144
Catterson, Gen. R. F., 35-37
Chambers, Gen. A., 9, 113, 124, 128, 137
Champion, Gen. T. E., 37-41
Chapman, Capt. E. D., 11, 114
Chase, Secretary S. P., 77
Chickering, Gen. T. E., 9, 119, 121, 129
Cholera, 92
Clary, Gen. R. E., 11
Commissary-General, Confederate, 87-89
Commitment to medicine, 147-148
Community leadership, 147, 159-160
Company officers, 4
Control enlistees, 8, 10, 11
Control generals, 8, 9
Control Groups, 8-13
Control surgeons, 10, 12
Cook, Lt. Col. T. Z., 11, 119, 126
Coolidge, Lt. Col. R. H., 12, 117, 146
Crawford, Gen. S. W., 13, 41-44, 72
Crimean war, 78, 100, 101
Crook, Gen. G., 9, 113, 119, 121, 133, 137
Crossing of paths, 134-135
Curtin, Gov. A., 66

D

Dandy, Gen. G. B., 6
Date, of birth, 105
  of discharge, 137
  of generalcy, 123-124

Davis, Jefferson, 15
Davis, Gen. R., 7
Dengue fever, 42
Dennison, Gov. W., 69, 78
Doan, Gen. A. W., 11
Duffee, Surg. J. H., 12, 117, 126, 140, 142
Duryee, Gen. J. E., 9, 119, 122
Dustin, Gen. D., 44-46
Duty as general officer prior to appointment, 124-125
Dysentery and diarrhea, 24, 31, 45, 62, 64, 71, 75, 83, 101, 103, 127, 128, 138, 146

E

Education,
from the war, 139-140
medical, 107, 147, 148-149
military, 112, 114
premedical, 106
postdoctoral, 107
Elliott, Gen. S. M., 46-48
Elliott, Gen. W. L., 6
Ellis, Gen. A. V., 9, 119, 126, 127
Elwell, Gen. J. J., 13, 48-50
Ely, Gen. R., 9
Erysipelas, 28, 67, 127
Evidence of prior medical education, 131-132

F

Father's occupation, 106
First South Carolina Regiment, 4
Freedman's Bureau, 25, 55, 93, 100, 125

G

Gano, Gen. R. M., 50-52, 63
Gans, Surg. G. C., 12, 126, 141
Gardner, Surg. P., 12, 121
Gardner, Gen. W. M., 9, 113, 130
Gates, Gen. T. B., 11, 114, 125
Generals,
Number, 5
medical corps, 5
prewar occupations, 165-167
state, 7
Gillespie, Capt. A., 11, 119
Gorgas, Gen. J., 11, 134, 144
Granbury, Gen. H. B., 11, 111, 114, 119, 126, 128
Grant, Gen. U. S., 27, 60, 63, 70, 71, 134
Grant, President, U. S., 71
Gray-Beard Regiment, 123
Gross, Dr. Samuel, 67, 81
Gwyn, Gen. J., 6

H

Hadlock, Lt. Col. W. E., 11, 118
Hamlin, Governor, 97, 113
Hammond, Surgeon-General W. A., 5
Hancock, Gen. W. S., 158
Hard, Surg. A., 12, 146
Harris, Gen. T. M., 52-56
Harrison, Surg. E. B., 12, 126, 142
Harrison, Pres. Benjamin, 45, 80, 98
Harrison, Pres. W. H., 168
Hartranft, Gen. J. F., 9, 110, 133, 144
Hayes, President R. B., 64, 80
Heinrichs, Gen. G., 11
Herrick, Surg. O. Q., 11, 141
Hickcox, Maj. E. J., 11, 119, 126
Hill, Surg. J. R., 12
Hillis, Gen. D. B., 56-58
Hillyer, Gen. W. S., 9, 119, 121, 122, 126, 129
Hood's Brigade of Texans, 89, 90, 91
Hurd, Surg. A., 12, 126, 142

I

Iowa Medical Journal, 109
Invalid Corps, 158

J

Jaundice, 28, 127, 128
Johnson, President Andrew, 55
Jones, Surg. J. C., 12, 140, 142, 143

K

Kiernan, Gen. J. L., 58-61, 74
Kimball, Surg. J. E. L., 12
Kimball, Gen. N., 51, 61-65, 72, 142
King, Gen. R., 9, 11, 111, 113, 119, 121, 122, 126, 130

Kinsman, Gen. J. B., 9, 121, 125
Kirkwood, Governor, 27, 57, 113

L

Leake, Gen. J. B., 9, 111, 119, 144
Leasure, Gen. D., 8, 65-68
Leggett, Gen. M. D., 68-72, 92, 93, 94
Length of military service, 118-120
Lincoln conspirators, 55
Lincoln, President A., 16, 62, 63, 65, 74
Lippincott, Gen. C. E., 73-76
Lippitt, Gen. F. J., 9, 110, 119, 121, 144
Logan, Gen. J. A., 9, 110, 111, 121, 133, 144
Longevity and death, 145-146
Ludlow, Gen. B. C., 76-78
Lyle, Gen. P., 9
Lyman, Lt. Col. G. H., 12, 114, 117, 140, 142, 143

M

Malaria, 15, 28, 60, 75, 95, 127, 128, 138, 146, 150
Manson, Gen. M. D., 6
Martin, Surg. C., 12, 109, 126
Matching enlistees, 8, 10, 11
McCormick, Dr. Charles, 150
McDermont, Lt. Col. C., 11, 112, 141, 144
McEwen, Gen. M., 117
McGugin, Surg. D. L., 12, 109, 110, 114, 126, 141, 142, 143, 146
McGuire, Surg. Hunter, 4
McMillen, Gen. W. L., 78-80
McNeil, Gen. J., 9, 110, 112, 121
McPheeters, Surg. J. G., 12, 126
Measles, 39, 44, 56, 83
Medical and other writing, 142-144
Medical Corps, generals, 5
Medical development, 147, 149-151
Medical education, 107, 147, 148-149
Medical Press, 59
Medical training by the war, 139-140
Meeker, Lt. Col. D., 12, 117, 140, 142, 143, 146
Meteorological service, 86
Mexican War, 15, 58, 62
Michler, Gen. N., 9, 113, 119, 121, 137, 144
Migration and travel, 111-112, 161-164
Milhau, Surg. J. J., 12, 112, 142
Military ambition, 147, 160-161
Military education and training, 112-114
Military efficiency and distinction, 132-134
Military medicine, 151-157
Miller, Gen. A. O., 81-84
Miller, Gen. M., 9, 110, 119
Moore, Surgeon-General, S. P., 3, 5, 12, 117, 142, 143
Morton, Gov. O. P., 62, 65
Multiple professions, 168-169
Myer, Gen. A. J., 13, 85-87, 127

N

Neal, Surg. T. S., 11, 118, 119, 141
Neff, Capt. A. J., 11, 118, 119, 126
Newhaus, Surg. C., 12, 126, 129
Newman, Surg. A., 12, 140, 142, 143
Nichols, Surg. H. W., 12
Northrop, Gen. L. B., 13, 87-89, 127
Norval, Lt. Col. J., 12, 117, 141

O

Occupations in addition to medicine, 108, 144-145
Officers, number, 4
Original medical and military contributions, 135-136
Original rank, 121-122
Osteomyelitis, 43

P

Page, Gen. R. L., 9, 113, 119, 121, 122, 144
Palmer, Surg. T. M., 12, 110, 114, 140, 141
Patrick, Gen. M. R., 6
Patriotism and belief in the cause, 147, 157-159
Pearce, Lt. J., 11, 119, 126
Perryman, Col. W. W., 11

Physician-soldiers, number, 3, 4
Physicians as field grade officers, 162-163, 164
Place of birth, 105, 112
Political interest and activity, 110
Porter, Col. A. B., 11, 119, 126
Postdoctoral education, 107
Premedical education, 106
Prewar medical practice, 108
Promotion despite disability, 129-130
Puerperal sepsis, 67, 68

Q

Quincy, Gen. S. M., 11

R

Ranks and grades, 116-118
Rathbone, Col. J. C., 11, 119
Reasons for choosing combatant service, 132, 147
Reeves, Surg. J. S., 12
Regimental officers, 4
Residual disease and disability, 137-139
Return to medicine and teaching, 140-142
Review of Medicine and Surgery, 78
Rex, Surg. G. P., 12, 109
Rheumatism, 28, 34, 55, 58, 127, 128, 138
Robertson, Gen. F. M., 91
Robertson, Gen. J. B., 63, 89-91
Roddey, Gen. P. D., 9, 110
Role of wounds and disease, 126-129
Rutherford, Gen. F. S., 11, 119, 126

S

Salter, Surg. R. H., 12, 126
Scott, Capt. F. G., 11, 119, 126
Scott, Gen. R. K., 91-94
Scurvy, 39, 83, 128, 131, 150
Searing, Col. W., 11
Service with Negro troops or Freedman's Bureau, 125-126
Sewell, Gen. W. J., 9, 112, 126, 128
Shepard, Surg. E. M., 12, 117, 141
Signal Corps, 86, 120
Smallpox, 72, 128, 131, 150
Smith, Lt. Col. D. P., 12, 117, 140, 141, 142, 143
Smith, Surg. J. P., 12, 117, 126
Speer, Lt. Col. A. M., 12, 117, 140, 142
Spirit of adventure, 161-164
Stanley, Gen. D. S., 6
Stanton, Secretary E. M., 64
Surgeons as casualties, 4
Sykes, Gen. G. W., 11, 114, 134

T

Tod, Governor, 78
Trail of death, Seventy-second Indiana, 83-84
Tuberculosis, 40, 127, 128, 138, 146, 150
Type of military service, 120-121
Typhoid fever, 44, 128

U

Udell, Surg. N., 12, 109, 110, 126, 142
Umbilical hernia, 70-71

W

Wagner, Gen. G. D., 11, 111
Wainwright, Gen. W. P., 94-96
Walcott, Gen. C. F., 9, 144
Ward, Col. G. T., 10, 11, 111, 118, 119, 126, 128
Warren, Gen. Joseph, 6
Welsh, Gen. W., 9, 121, 122, 125, 137
Wentworth, Gen. M. F., 96-99
Wild, Gen. E. A., 99-101
Wild's African Brigade, 100
Willard, Surg. J. N., 11, 119, 126, 141
Williams, Gen. D. H., 9, 119, 144
Wilson, Surg. A., 12

Y

Yandell, Dr. D. Y., 52, 81
Yates, Governor R., 73
Yellow fever, 42, 49, 127, 150

Z

Zinn, Gen. G., 9, 122, 128
Zulich, Gen. S. M., 8, 101-104